Be Health Beautiful

Use Great Nutrition to Gain Control of Your Life

CARISSA KRETSCHMER, HOLISTIC NUTRITIONAL COUNSELOR

Thank you Achim, for your incredible support of all of my thoughts and ideas. Thank you for being my rock and my biggest fan. Thank you, my dear sweet husband, for being in our lives with your perfect heart and every drop of your soul.

Thank you Nicky, for being so beautiful in your heart and for your ever-overflowing optimism. I love you, my dear sweet son.

Thank you, Jamie. You hold the bar high for us to reach for in our lives. Your humor and wit, coupled with your openness to beautiful things, is a wonderful inspiration. I love you.

Achim, Nicky, and Jamie, I love you for eating the food that I prepare for you and for understanding that my love for you is truly what makes me whole. You are all Healthy and Beautiful, and you are my inspiration to keep helping the rest of the world to become as beautiful as you are.

Contents

Acknowledgements

I would like to recognize the scientific community for their ongoing contributions in the area of nutrition, disease and biology. I am grateful to the researchers and their peers who analyze data, work by stringent ethical standards, and bring their findings to our attention through scientific publications. You are my heroes.

Achim Kretschmer, my accountability partner during this writing process. When I could not see the words and needed the eye of someone who knows how I think and what I wanted to say, he was my dictionary, thesaurus, grammar inspector, and technical advisor, all of which he can add to a long list of notable accomplishments. THANK YOU!

My editor, Allison M. Sidhu, who was extraordinary with her suggestions and questions that allowed my message to be thoroughly expressed. Allison kept me very busy and eloquently supported the integrity of my work. Thank you for pushing me and bringing out the best parts of the message of this book. My gratitude is honest and heartfelt.

Liza Schklar, the graphic designer responsible for this beautiful cover. You heard my words and granted my wish to express with an image what being Health Beautiful is all about. Thank you, Liza.

.

My Story of Food and Body

The beginning of my story as I remember it was first told to me by my mother: I was always an allergic child. I was allergic to milk, soy, rice, meat, and all preservatives. I was born in 1970, so there were preservatives in every type of packaged food. Packaged food was promoted and regarded during this era as the best way to feed your family.

I remember lying on the floor of the upstairs landing with my siblings surrounding me. I remember feeling dizzy and outside of myself. I was only three years old at the time of that first incident. I could not relate to the bodily sensations that I was experiencing. I could not regain normal feelings in my limbs. I could not breathe deeply. I was very dizzy, and scared, very scared. An ambulance was called and the paramedics used oxygen and fluids to revive me.

Because there were six of us in the family, we obviously had done and eaten many different things. My parents could not put their finger on what was happening to me. The idea that food could have this effect on my health was far from everyone's minds. Today this way of thinking has changed—the prospect of allergies is what we head to first for answers. It took several incidences of the same weird feeling I had felt on the stairs before we were finally able to identify food as the culprit.

My godmother was the one to conclude that I might have an allergy to milk and preservatives. She is an Italian woman who comes from a family that cooks, and she relates to food on an organic level. She had five of her own children and was thinking practically, not medically. This is not to say that my parents weren't home cooks; they were just relying on the good doctor's word. They were likely thinking, as many do today, *certainly our food couldn't be harming our daughter*. This concept became something that has always stayed with me, and I see it in my practice every day. Food, the very thing that we cannot avoid for the purposes of survival– is this what makes so many get sick and die? I realize now the enormous effect the discovery of my reactions to certain foods had on me throughout my life.

After the several ambulance calls and near-death episodes, my mother went back to serving real, unprocessed food cooked from scratch in our home. She would pin notes to my shirt when I went to new places on my own that read "Do Not Feed This Child." I was isolated in this way. I remember going to a live taping of "The Uncle Al Show" as an audience member when cookies were distributed to the children. They were the chocolate flower-shaped kind, with sugar sprinkled on top. As all the children were eating, a stagehand came over to me and took my cookie away saying, "Your mother said you cannot have this."

I knew why. I knew that it could kill me. I was about five then, and I just did not have a true grasp on how harmful it really could be for me to eat a food that had been prepared with god knows what. I am sure it was a bad-tasting cookie, certainly not up to my standards today, but as a kid at a television show taping, all I wanted was to be able to eat that cookie. It was the seventies and food allergies were just not as prevalent as they are today. Over time, I realized that I do not have food allergies. What happens to me is a severe reaction to the chemicals that are added to certain foods as preservatives, additives and fillers. I can thank my childhood experience for setting the foundation for my career today. It was a matter of life or death for me as a child, but food is really a matter of life or death for everyone.

I know the negative feeling that I have towards drugs and alcohol today is attributed to that feeling of being outside and out of control of my own body. Today I do not like feeling drunk. I never liked feeling drugged. I have always felt trapped in circumstances where I could not control the situation. It's no wonder that I feel this way. Can you imagine being a baby and feeling drugged, without the words to express it or any sense of understanding as to what was happening? No adult could explain it to me adequately for a long while, and the very fact that it was food that was killing me is in itself frightening. I *did* understand that food can be dangerous if it is manipulated in certain ways.

Processed food became the thing I knew to avoid at all costs. Today it is the same. I don't need an ambulance nearby if I consume milk, soy or preservatives, but I avoid all processed food. The processed food chain begins with how an animal or animal product that a person consumes is raised. For example, I take extra measures to ensure that the eggs that I eat come from pasture-raised chickens that are fed a vegetarian soy-free diet, because I feel sick if I eat eggs that come from chickens that have been fed soy.

In adolescence, I would eat fast food and junk food frequently. I tried to be that kid at the television show taping who could eat the cookie, but it never worked. Although I would eat these foods to fit in and be part of the adolescent crowd, I would still feel sick and uncomfortable, and displayed symptoms of food intolerances. The self-destructive behavior was compounded by my adolescent view of my body and a lack of confidence. In addition to the physical rejection of these foods, I also viewed my body's appearance in a very critical way. I, like many girls, struggled with my body image. A lot of my upbringing was about being tiny. The girls in my family danced ballet and the teachers were brutal to my sister. She has a full figure but this is just not an acceptable part of the ballet world. I always wanted to be thinner. I always felt the need to show my best figure in every outfit. I would change my clothes many times before finally finding an outfit that I was happy with. I can honestly say I was like that until very recently.

As I gained control of my health through food choices that serve me, I've gained confidence and wisdom. Today I am very thin and strong. It is not an obsession any longer because I have finally applied what I learned as a sick kid to my actual body. Real food cooked with love and from scratch makes a healthy, slim, strong person. That is how I hope to educate my clients and my readers. If you take one thing from this book, let it be that nutritious food will help you to create a balance between your inner health and outward appearance, where you are at the perfect size, weight, and state of health.

I am finicky about what I eat. I won't just eat anything or purchase my food from anywhere. My standards are high. For instance, when I shop for vegetables, I go to a market where I can count on finding vibrantly colored, fresh vegetables. I never just grab the first one I see. Instead, I hand-select each, checking for firmness, fragrance and where and how it was grown. This will ensure that my meal will deliver the greatest flavor and quality that I can provide for myself and my family. And why not? I wish more people had high food standards. Then there would be more healthy restaurant choices and all supermarkets, large and small, would offer the highest quality food as common fare.

I grew into adulthood investing more effort into assuring the quality of my food, experimenting with technical recipes that required me to hunt down elusive and expensive ingredients such as saffron and lavender extract. While it was very exciting to execute these kinds of recipes, some required various types of sausages or foie gras that had a negative effect on my health.

In the last twenty years I have traveled to Europe almost every year, visiting my husband's family. I tried to eat meat and cream-based foods and tried to embrace the culture of eating meat for breakfast, lunch and dinner, and then attempted to solve the resulting digestive unrest with high percentage aperitifs before and after meals. I had a passion for experiencing and sharing in these gourmet delights and I wanted to cook and share these meals with my friends. As I developed a cognitive approach to eating, I've been able to enjoy the beauty of exotic foods while making selections that support my health. It is possible to find high quality and healthy food anywhere. It is a matter of letting your health be a priority over the fashionable trends of the moment.

I didn't always eat high-end gourmet meals. I tried to drink juices made with aspartame and artificially colored and flavored foods. They all disgusted me. I would gag when I tried to eat them, ending up doubled over on the sofa after meals. I would take a small taste of boxed lemonade and spit it out with a "Yuck! How can someone drink this stuff? It's awful." I developed a keen taste bud sensation over the years, and I believe I can taste the more subtle ingredients in food. My husband said I would make an incredible wine taster. I can distinguish the most subtle flavors in a dish. I realize this is a survival tactic for me. Like taking a poison and tasting the bitterness, I can consume a food and taste the chemicals that were used to make it.

It is no wonder that I am a finicky eater. I have a high bar when it comes to where and what I will let pass my lips. I love to cook. I no longer have to worry about what I am eating or what hidden ingredient may have adverse effects on me. I love to eat. I am in touch with food and how it relates to my body. I share food with everyone, and everyone loves my cooking. My friends are often surprised at how simple it is to make what I cook. I cook in a simple way without a lot of ingredients, with just a few spices, made with basic kitchen appliances. This I know for sure: my food is great, because I use fresh herbs and high quality pure ingredients, which allow amazing flavor to come through in finished dishes. Today my body is in excellent health, and my words to you are the truth. Real food is the key to health.

Be Amazing

Vitality and vigor are qualities that I want for my family and myself. That is why I try to never let my family down when it comes to food. I know it is the most basic and lasting contribution that I can give to them. Every person has biological needs that are met through nutritional information found in their food. Every time I give my family highly nutritious meals, I understand that I supplied their bodies with food that will support their health. By supporting their health with nutritional food, my family can face their individual challenges and the demands that their days require of them.

My children don't have to worry about becoming sluggish or experiencing sugar drops when they need energy the most. I give them a consistent supply of beneficial food that supports cognitive health, which allows them to achieve academic success. I understand how a constant source of various nutritional information, such as protein and calcium, becomes depleted and needs to be replenished throughout the day. A replenishment of such elements supports their growing bones and strong muscles, and leads them to be powerful individuals. What I want for my family more than anything is their happiness, and I know in my heart as well as my head that a healthy existence is a happy one.

I have posed the question, "What is your legacy?" to seminar groups and my social network community. Many sweet and poetic replies have been expressed in response to my question. Motivational speaker Eric Thomas once asked this of his audience. He was aiming to get each individual to question who and what he or she is today. He wanted his audience to act in a way that would help them to achieve their envisioned legacies. In many cases, you will be known for what your actions are while you are alive.

I can honestly say that I conduct my life in ways that will allow me to leave a legacy that I can be proud of. I understand that although I strive to become the person who I look up to, and although I struggle with things that are hard for me, I always strive to do the best I can with the actions that I have control over. I know that when I make a choice to eat something, it will be the best possible food that I can get. My family can count on me to protect their health relentlessly. I can stand toe-to-toe with any nutritional challenge and I will come out on top.

Eric Thomas will tell you that hard work will pay out in life above all else. When something comes easily to a person, they won't have a realistic understanding of how valuable that skill is to their ultimate success. When I get up early in the morning and set my goals for the day, I know in my heart that I will try my hardest to meet each one of those goals. I understand that by striving to hit my goals every day, I can look forward to celebrating accomplishments both large and small. Setting goals and meeting them is extremely rewarding. That is why I look forward to this process in my daily life. You can live the life you want by taking control of the simplest necessities. Serving your nutritional needs every day has rewarding payouts throughout your life. Setting the goal to nourish your body and become Health Beautiful will lead you to success in work, family, relationships and finding happiness. Taking control of your health strengthens and powers your body to function with peak performance outcomes. Being the person who protects your body and honors these needs will enrich it with love and passion for living that goes beyond your dreams.

Setting out to write this book was an incredibly challenging goal on multiple levels. The logistics of finding balance between work, family and my personal life taxed me every day; having fulfilled such a huge dream that was so challenging to me rewarded every aspect of my being. I set my mind on making this goal happen and now it is in your hands.

One of the things I'm most proud of is having the ability to strike a balance in my day-to-day life, even when I'm faced with crises and fulfilling the demands of challenging goals. Supporting my physical health is my secret weapon for taking control of my life. Taking control of my health allowed me to reach for dreams that I never thought possible. Food has always been a part of my life and the study of biology has always been a passion of mine. I've had to uncover what I needed in my physical being to discover my potential. My health is my purpose. My personal health has given me the ability to heal others and to coach people towards successful, fulfilling lives. The actions that I have taken to regain control of my health have enabled me to enjoy the luxury of success.

Taking control of your health will do the same for you. Stop settling into the life of a drone, living with the madness of exhaustion and sickness. Don't accept the health bumps in your road as unmovable. Reach for greatness. Set a goal to be healthy right now. Don't live with pain and insomnia. Don't just accept weight gain as a part of aging. Make the decision to love yourself enough to give yourself every possible chance to be amazing.

Health Beautiful The Lifestyle

A lifestyle is something that is your norm, the everyday instinctual response that you have to every moment of your life. You don't second guess the choices you make, whether selecting food, deciding where to shop, choosing where to work out, or selecting your preferred style of clothing. This also includes where you choose to live and how you decide to design and decorate your home. Your lifestyle is also comprised of how you drive to work and the approach that you take towards enjoyment, whether you like going to the movies, concerts, or dinners out, and whether you prefer vacationing on cruises or in cities.

The Health Beautiful lifestyle resides in an upper echelon. The person who is Health Beautiful does not enjoy poor quality food, nor would she allow junk food to pass her lips. If she needs a sweet treat, she demands and deserves the very best, the one item that is truly what a Health Beautiful person desires and not just any old dusty candy bar off the shelf.

You can enjoy the best that life has to offer– it is often just a matter of allowing yourself to have it. Higher quality food will improve your quality of health just like a more comfortable bed will help you to attain better sleep. Allowing yourself more time for enjoyment will lead to a more enjoyable life.

You are Better Than a Circus Peanut

I have a dear friend who always jokes with me about trying the junkiest food available. She and I banter about what I will allow into my world. Since we were young adults sitting outside the convenience store, when she introduced me to prepackaged cakes colored hot pink and filled with foamy cream, we have laughed about how disgusted I am, and how amazed I am by the so-called food that is sold and that people actually eat every day.

Once we were at a concert with a large group of women when she pulled out some circus peanuts. It was almost like a dare: Will Carissa eat such a thing? Nope! I told everyone that I am better than a circus peanut. It was quite funny and now this is a catchphrase that we use often: "Don't eat that, you are better than a circus peanut!" And for goodness sake, don't give it to your kids.

Put your Head in the Game

The gist of this little story is to raise your personal bar when it comes to food. I invite you now to discard the old, once-acceptable prepackaged food that supermarkets and large food producers push on you through advertising. I encourage you now to set a standard that encourages you to purchase and consume the highest quality food available to you every day. Choose the fresh fruit that looks the plumpest, smells the fruitiest, and feels the firmest, because only the freshest and fruitiest items are the ones that provide you with the highest energy possible.

Let's say it is January and you go to the produce aisle. You look around and it's likely that oranges are the most colorful item available. That is because oranges are a winter fruit. Eating seasonally is highly beneficial, it is cost effective, and it incorporates the best quality and most energy-packed food into your diet. Seasonal eating is an example of elevating your food standards as part of a Health Beautiful lifestyle. While you can get oranges here in New York in the summer, they couldn't compare to the taste and quality of an orange that you would select during the winter season. The same goes for many different kinds of produce. When selecting an orange in season, a Health Beautiful person would choose firm oranges with a tight skin and a light, orangey fragrance. The Health Beautiful individual hand selects each orange and never buys a large presorted bag of fruit. Being selective and looking for excellence in your food is one of the ways to ensure high quality in your food.

Seasonal eating will propel your health forward easily. The quality and taste of fresh produce is unmatched when compared to what large chain supermarkets offer. A gardener knows instinctively when their fruit is ready for harvest. They may brush the leaves and smell to see if a fragrance is released, or they will have developed a particular touch to see if the perfect tenderness appears on their vegetables and fruit. Although most of us don't grow our own oranges, you can develop a keen sense of the ripeness and freshness of your food, discounting the visual appearance and not being swayed by wax-covered, shiny fruit or pre-packaged produce.

The Health Beautiful person eats oranges in the winter along with all kinds of citrus. Eating oranges that contain seeds is fine– messy but good. In winter you also want to eat lemons and other types of citrus like grapefruit and Meyer lemons. You should be cooking with these fruits and using them on your salads in addition to eating whole oranges, grapefruit and other types of citrus.

Seasonal fruit has a way of creating a rhythm in your body similar to your sleep rhythms. We develop eating rhythms and can draw from the season what we need to be balanced in our lives. Eating citrus, which grows in high places, lifts your energy and spirits. It brightens and lifts the flavors of your food as well. Eating root vegetables, also in season during the winter, will root and ground your spirits, providing earthy flavor to your food. The two, root vegetables and citrus, grow in opposing places, offering a perfectly balanced compliment to each other in your food and in your body. The bright citrus brightens while we are indoors all winter and the root vegetables ground us with comfort to keep us warm.

Let me take a minute to discuss juice versus whole fruit. I often talk about chewing your food rather than drinking your food. Your body is designed to chew as a part of the digestive process. Foods like oranges have fiber that gets broken down throughout the digestive process. Your body looks to process its own food by forming bonds, using enzymes and various chemicals to absorb nutrients from whole food. The digestive process is complex and each step is purposeful and beneficial to your overall health.

Eating an orange whole is always preferred to juicing an orange. Your teeth and saliva work to start the digestive process of breaking down the fiber in the orange. Your digestive enzymes are activated and bonds are created that permit a slow uptake of the sugar in an orange, all while converting the vitamins into information that your body will use. Through the activation of a slow digestion of fiber and fructose, your blood sugar will not spike rapidly as it does when you are drinking fiber-free juice. Chewing and eating the orange enables an active metabolic process to take place.

When you drink a glass of orange juice, the body feels refreshed at first and thirst is temporarily quenched. Without the fiber found in the whole orange, the sugar in the juice is rapidly absorbed into your bloodstream. Elevated blood sugar triggers a response in the body to regulate the imbalance. Insulin is released from the pancreas and blood pressure rises because of the demands being put on your organs. Drinking juice creates the same responses in the body as drinking a large glass of soda. Drinking sugary beverages like orange juice, other types of juice and soda on a regular basis calls on the body to constantly react to elevated sugar in the blood. The constant need for insulin release can result in pancreatic exhaustion.

Pancreatic exhaustion is when the pancreas can no longer produce the proper amount of insulin needed to process high blood sugar levels. It often results in type 2 diabetes. There is a vast amount of scientific literature that I encourage you to read for a fuller understanding of what is happening to you if you indeed have been diagnosed with type 2 diabetes. The pre-diabetic people who have come to me seeking nutritional guidance have all been warned by their doctors to stay away from sugary beverages.

One simple way to avoid disease is to chew your food.

Developing a sense of quality and satisfaction in eating whole food sets you up for proper digestion and ease in your body's responses to the food that you supply to it. Don't start your children on a path of elevated blood sugar and the need to constantly produce insulin in their little bodies. Juice sold in containers is not a healthy option for anyone. Rather than choosing a sugary juice box, offer yourself and your kids a ripe, seasonal, fragrant, satisfying and beneficial piece of fruit instead.

The costs and nutritional benefits of eating whole fruit are also reflected in preparing your own dishes at home. I can make guacamole in less than five minutes and it is wholesome and delicious. In contrast, when I have looked at the packaging on guacamole dips in the supermarket and read the ingredients, well... yuck! The unhealthy ingredients that manufacturers put in that package are not only bad for your health on so many levels, they are also overpriced and totally unnecessary. I have seen added sugar, corn syrup, and artificial preservatives on these labels. No wonder it can stay on the shelf so long—it is a chemical mixture of garbage! My homemade guacamole lasts for just one sitting for two reasons: First, it is so good there is nothing left over for another day, and second, because the only "preservative" I use is lime juice.

By raising the lifestyle bar and making your own food at home, you are able to save money while altering your personal tastes. When you are constantly feeding yourself foods that contain corn-based preservatives, your palate becomes adapted to increasingly sweet sensations, and more added sugar and artificial ingredients are required to satisfy your tastes. Mark Hyman, an American physician, scholar and New York Times best-selling author and founder of the UltraWellness Center, refers to this as a hyper palatable state.[1] Dr. Hyman speaks of this and writes about this state in his books and lectures. Food producers make sweeter and sweeter food, which you then need to eat more and more of to feel satisfied. The fat and sickness accumulates while the food producers make more and more money. Stop the cycle here. You deserve fresh, high quality food. Make these choices with each item on your plate.

Start by selecting only what you will be able to eat within four days when you make your choices at the grocery store. Do not overwhelm yourself with large volumes of prepackaged food, even if it is on sale. The large package of discounted food is not going to last longer than the homemade food, and if it does it will likely be thrown out later anyway. This is a common complaint and stressor among big box store shoppers. They buy too much and lug it home just to throw half of it out in one week's time. In order to keep such large quantities on the shelves, the harvest-to-table timeframe is long, leaving the flavor diminished and the quality undesirable. A great deal of produce, such as tomatoes, are harvested before they are properly and naturally ripened. The produce is then packaged and sold to the consumer many days later. Wilted and sometimes even moldy pieces are often found hidden among the fresher bits in a large package of food. Flavor and ripeness are more easily selected by the consumer who buys food in smaller quantities.

It is important to wean yourself off of the massive amounts of food that are always available in your kitchen at all times. Purchasing large quantities of food at one time is a huge cost, and bringing it home, unpacking it and putting it all away is a time consuming task. One tub of guacamole found at a warehouse-style supermarket was approximately $9 at the time of publication of this book. The package of guacamole that I found contains ten ingredients, most of which are meant to act as flavoring and preservatives, two things that are added to prepared and packaged foods that can contribute to unwanted weight gain. Homemade guacamole costs me approximately $4 to make three to four servings, and I will not have to have a huge party in order to get my money's worth.

Homemade items will also aid in promoting your health,

rather than taking away from your health. Your body is looking for information, found in the food that you eat, to perform properly. We want to eat food that tastes amazing and fulfills our needs. Creating homemade meals using high quality ingredients with the best possible natural flavor is not only desired by a healthy individual, but satisfies the nutritional needs for maintaining good health as well. Developing the instinct to recognize great quality food that supports excellent health is an instinct that Health Beautiful people enjoy.

You Need to Want it More Than You Want to Breathe

Lifestyle includes all aspects of your day. Money and the lack of money tend to cause a stalling effect in people's lives. The lack of money can cause someone to be consumed with worry about bills and the ability to provide for their family. Some people will use eating out or drinking or smoking as crutches that give them a much needed break from reality. I am not speaking from an ivory tower when I attempt to lead you toward breaking these habits. I have lived in those places and I am not immune to temptation or defeat. It is because of my well-worn path that I know how to overcome the self-depravation, and it is this journey that has led me and my family to raise our standards, and to uphold standards that are high. It is a matter of knowing what you need, and understanding what is good for you and what is bad for you.

It is important to remain focused on how great you feel when you eat a healthy meal or take a brisk walk or love someone with a whole heart. Because of this, I encourage you to examine how you want to feel, look, and be in your everyday life. Years ago, I spent a lot of my time focusing on how I didn't like how I looked in my clothes. This is typical for women everywhere, right? The change came when I switched my focus to wanting to recapture how I felt during my healthiest moments.

I was on a hike, doing quite well, walking briskly with my dog and feeling really good, when I came to another hiker three times my age. His pace was just as brisk and he looked amazing. He told me about his sick wife and how she couldn't walk with him due to severe complications of sciatica. Yet there he was, about eighty, hiking the same trail as me with love in his eyes and a great attitude in spite of his trials.

I realized then that my health had nothing to do with how I looked or who was with me, or how much money I had or didn't have in my bank account. I realized then that I can aspire to be eighty-plus years old, hiking on a nature trail with a dog and nothing but my own body powering me forward. That was the moment when I decided to forget the bulging bra strap line, forget the bills, forget the media, and forget the people who were not walking with me on my path toward health. I had to acknowledge that I was the only person who could make my legs walk and feed my body and nourish my soul with what it needed to become Health Beautiful.

This is the secret to success in everything you do: You need to want it more than you want to breathe. You need to want your health for you, and not anyone else but you. All the rest will be bonuses in a great life. Wanting great health so that you are not a burden on your kids is not enough to inspire you to always make the right choices to support your health. This is because you know deep inside that someone will probably take care of you regardless of how you lived thirty years prior. The people taking care of you when you are old won't say, "No, you ate a donut in 2015 so I won't care for you now." Wanting to avoid being a burden is a poor motivator. Weight and body image are terrible motivators too, because of the phenomenon known as morphed body image. That is where you see yourself as an ugly being regardless of how positively others see you.

Here is where I want you to grab control of your own life. Maybe hikes aren't your favorite thing and that is okay, that is my thing. It is up to you to find your thing. I found motivation from the healthy elder community: my grandmother, my hiking friend, the woman who takes Dance Jam classes at the gym and wears sequined tops and knee-high leg warmers at age 70. I take motivation from intelligent people who mindfully select food and restaurants, who are not just moving with the masses towards big chain restaurants that pile too much food too high on their customers' plates. I take my motivation from taking on activities that I have not yet mastered, like meditation. I have a lot of trouble clearing my mind and sitting still. I know that when I need to be calm, I wish that I could have this in my bag of tricks to utilize. Some people look to me for motivation because I am so disciplined in my food and exercise habits. I am motivated by being a leader or a role model. I am not just responsible for my own wellbeing, but also the wellbeing of many people around me.

Being Health Beautiful is not about letting life happen to you, but rather, actively making greatness a main part of your life. Greatness resides in a place where you deliver more than average outcomes to the world. Whatever feeds that desire for greatness will be your *why,* your purpose, a vision of the person that you want to be in the world. Your reason for needing to be healthy motivates the ways in which you are able to continue to make great choices in your life. It will enable the people that you love and the world around you to count on your actions to inspire and protect them. The reason that you have selected this book and decided to make the changes that will make you Health Beautiful will form your core beliefs and your focus.

Taking the reins of your life and steering yourself towards excellent health will result in the achievement of control. Clarity in discovering why you make the choices that you make throughout your day is easy to discover when you approach the day with great health. Being hungry and tired or fog-brained and sick makes it difficult to deal with everyday responsibilities. Stress comes at everybody all day and keeps many people up all night. Stress is more easily managed when your heart rate is not always elevated, or when you're not dealing with nutritional deficiencies.

Perhaps aiming to manage your stress is your reason for

deciding to improve your health. Perhaps being able regain intimacy with your partner is why you want to be healthy. Your reasons may not be clear all at once. That is part of the process of discovering your purpose. Looking for your reasons for great health and focusing on why you need to be healthy begins with a desire that sparks a need for greatness in your life. Wanting excellent health in a way that's just as strong as your need to breathe will keep you strong and focused on your successful journey through your Health Beautiful life.

Life is Already Happening- Time to Join

It is exciting to embark on new paths in life. Think about how exciting it is to plan a vacation or an evening out. We search for and plan the things that will bring us joy and make us feel happy. Making changes to your lifestyle to improve your health is a similar event. You are able to envision yourself looking a certain way and feeling happy. You get to experience new foods and try new activities.

I love to congratulate my new clients with a warm welcome and a celebration of their decision to take their health to a beautiful place. We strategize about ways to incorporate new activities into their routine and together we clarify their goals and plan paths for them to use in making their goals a reality. I give them a personalized journal to aid in setting daily goals and checking in each evening to see how they met their goals for the day. Over time, the person is able to change what they used to do into what serves their needs and satisfies their goals. The journal establishes direct links between what they want in their lives and how they plan to make those things happen.

The clients who use the journal find themselves reaching higher and further-reaching goals more easily than those who don't use it. They are able to establish how to get what they need to reach their daily goals. Breaking old habits that do not serve specific needs is a great deal easier when a written declaration is made early in the day. Examples of daily goals that my clients have written in their journals read like this: "I will give myself energy by feeding my body sunflower seeds; I will give myself love by taking a power walk during my break at two o'clock; I will provide myself with strength by eating salmon for dinner and working out using weights at four o'clock."

At the evening check-in, in they can look to see where they supported their needs and how their specific goals made them feel at the end of the day. As they rid themselves of bad habits and are feeling fulfilled later through the use of good choices, they begin to connect feeling great with serving their needs. Planning to do something that makes you happy and feeling happy as a result of achieving this is cause for celebration. As you learn to celebrate the accomplishments that brought you joy, you will discover how wonderful it is to be in control of your life using nutrition.

Take this as an example of living your life in the present while planning for your future. Your life is not happening later, it is happening now. You can't put it on hold. Why wait to be a part of it? Maybe your excuse is that you are overscheduled now and it doesn't seem like there is time to be active. That is an excuse that leaves control of your life in the hands of a schedule that adheres to outside demands and neglects your personal time and state of wellbeing. The very act of incorporating personal and physical activity time into your daily schedule is a healthy step towards gaining control of your life.

There is time for what you really want; it is just a matter of figuring out what that thing is that you want, and then taking it. Here are some ways to get started until you uncover your very own motivation for your healthy life. Motivation experts will often ask you to make one-, five- and ten-year plans for the future. I'd like you to start in the future and go backwards instead. Picture yourself at age eighty-five. What are you doing in every moment of every day? Ask yourself: Where will I live, and what does my home look like? How do I spend my mornings, afternoons and evenings? Who do I spend my time with? What do they love about me? What is my legacy at this point in my life? Now do the same for yourself at seventy-five years old, asking the same questions and examining the various aspects of who loves you, what your life looks like, and why. How do you spend your days and which moments do you look forward to living? Now do the same exercise for ages sixty-five, fifty-five, forty-five and so on until you get to your current age.

This exercise creates a motivational vision that is more authentic, because people will often describe a life that others expect of them rather than the life that they want to be living when the task is done in reverse. I have always felt uncomfortable looking ahead at my career. I felt conflicted with what I should want to aspire toward versus what I need to fulfill my dreams. I hear similar sentiments from my clients. They are afraid to look forward and are more comfortable looking back, so I start them way ahead in life and ask them to look back on what led them to where they ended up.

Have you ever said, "Tomorrow, I start a new diet and I will take control of my compulsive eating"? If so, you are among the majority of people. In the beginning of making true lifestyle changes, it is very important to be your own best friend. Don't let yourself down by giving in because of a lack of structure. Life is not structured into perfect lunch-sized healthy portions. We make our lives that way with tight schedules, relying on meals found in packages and takeout containers rather than making meals lovingly at home with healthy ingredients. We adhere to other people's demands and sidestep our personal responsibility to our own health. Just as the kids go to school at a certain time and you have to be at work at a certain time each day, or you have to make an appointment at a certain time, you need to structure your food schedule in ways that allow you to be healthy. The sad fact is that most food that is conveniently available, such as takeout Chinese food or canned ravioli for the kids, is junk food. You need to know where to look.

Grocery stores are an excellent go-to place for healthy fast food. You're almost always able to find cut up fresh fruit, and most stores have a health food section where you can get peanut butter (or other nut and seed butters), an apple and some hardboiled eggs. You'll find sushi, packages of seeds and nuts, whole grain salads, and dairy-free soups.

Snack choices can have different intended effects for different people. For a client who was looking to gain muscle mass, I recommended switching his snacks from chips and Tootsie Rolls to a bag of baby spinach and sunflower seeds. When he changed his habit from a quick dose of sugar to long-lasting healthy fat and vitamin-packed snacks, he had more energy and was able to lift heavier weights and bulk up as a result. For people wanting to get thin, certain clients restricted calories and ate a small yogurt for breakfast; however, I recommend natural oatmeal with sunflower seeds for breakfast and plain unsweetened yogurt as a post-workout snack. These meals will give them the energy to do lean cardio-driven exercise and repair and rebuild their muscles with good sources of protein. I always say I am skinny because of the way I eat; I look good in a bathing suit because of the way I work out. There is a big difference.

When you are on the go, keep an eye out for high quality food that can be prepared on the spot.

- I like Japanese restaurants for seaweed salad and steamed veggie rolls (not deep fried shrimp rolls)

- I love Whole Foods for soups and roasted vegetables

I never go to a supermarket and get anything that's labeled gluten free, sugar free, or fat free– these are metabolic killers. Fat-free translates to the replacement of fat with more sugar. Gluten-free means the replacement of pulverized, nutritionally stripped wheat flour with nutritionally stripped, pulverized grains that don't contain gluten. The substitute for sugar is artificial chemical sugar substitute, which has never been scientifically proven to aid in weight loss.

The removal or substitution of ingredients is not necessarily an indication of a healthy or health-promoting product.

Often it is just a way to sell you the product. A striking example is when companies label their bottled water gluten free. This label is ridiculous– all water is gluten free, but labeling it that way draws the consumer into buying this particular water over another brand. More effective food choices would be the ones that do not require a label, like whole fruit and vegetables. These unprocessed foods simply do not require such labels.

At all times, keep a container of very healthy snacks at hand that offer antioxidants and energy to hold you over between meals. I like to keep nuts, seeds and dark chocolate in the car. They keep well, and are fast recovery foods for me and my family to utilize after workouts and games or on long trips. People who begin this practice are able to have better self-control when they do get a chance to eat a proper meal. The clients who use this tactic make their own combinations of trail mix. This starts a practice of being prepared and meeting your needs before your hunger becomes a desperate situation. (If you are allergic to nuts or chocolate, find seeds instead, like sunflower and pumpkin seeds with sea salt.)

Bring your lunch and eat your breakfast

The reality is that if you don't eat, you will become hungry eventually. You wake and consume a caffeine-laden drink and, lo and behold, you have no appetite; that is the caffeine talking. You need to eat breakfast at the start of your day, preferably within the first hour after you wake. Eating breakfast early initiates a steady flow of nutrition and hydration to your body. It allows you to think and work at your full potential. The body will begin to rely on breakfast as a steady nutrient source and release energy according to this input. You need to hydrate early and chew food that's high in vitamins and carbohydrates in order to get though the day. Food is meant to fuel your action for the day.

You won't get thin from skipping breakfast and you won't get skinny from starvation. Eventually you will need to eat and eventually your body will start to shut down, creating health dilemmas. Starvation for the sake of controlling your impulses or in an effort to break bad eating habits complicates your weight loss attempts. A healthy way to start your day is to include energy-rich and hydrating foods into your morning routine. Acknowledge that you just went through an eight-hour fast from food and water while you slept. Rehydrating and introducing food back into your body soon after you wake is essential for your metabolism.

Every function that goes on in your body requires water. Whole berries are naturally filled with water and antioxidants. When my clients are starting to introduce breakfast to their routine, I recommend that they wake and start consuming berries as they go about their morning activities. Within a few days, this habit leads to making and eating more substantial, healthy and fortifying breakfasts. Having fortified their morning, they are better equipped, which leads to better food choices throughout the day. Your body wants and needs nutritious food to function.

Knowing what you need to achieve excellence in your day will help you to make positive decisions that will serve your specific requirements. Taking time to look at yourself and your day's requirements will be an empowering exercise for you. You will be able to reject food labels that are there simply to draw on weaknesses or impulses, meant to confuse and distract you from your main mission. The need to be healthy requires honest introspection about what you are doing to deprive yourself of beneficial nutrition. While starvation is easy for some people, they eventually find that the complications that result from not eating are far worse than simply getting real food into their diets to replace the junk. Buying food that is not giving your body the very best possible nutrients on a reliable schedule will only create negative consequences that impact your performance. Your health is about more than eating a vegetable and some fruit; it is about educating yourself about how food works and what your food does to make you a healthy individual.

Reject what you think is untrue when it comes to diet. This misinformation usually is made up by corporations who want to sell you something that will make you spend money (i.e. fat free, gluten free, sugar free, dairy free, 90-calorie yogurt, etc.), leading you to struggle until you eventually give it up in total frustration and go back to what you knew to be true in the first place.

Sleep for Your Health

A few key things are required for a healthy body: sleep, exercise, nourishment, and avoiding toxic scenarios as much as possible.

Sleep is a necessary part of being healthy. During sleep, the body recovers from the day's workout. Whether it is mental or physical, the body must have rest. Achieving restful sleep is a challenge for so many people today and I want to acknowledge the fact that everyone sleeps differently. Some sleep hard and heavy, then light and fitfully. Some hit the pillow and don't wake until eight hours later. Some lay awake, endlessly striving for sleep. Insomnia is a painful experience and I do not want to sugarcoat it with quick remedies. True insomniacs are desperate for quality sleep and will go to any end to find it. I urge those who cannot sleep well to look at the following aspects of your life, and see where you may be lacking or overcompensating.

Sleep does not need to occur in a sedated state. Drugs that cause you to sleep are designed to create a state of unconsciousness, and an inability to wake easily. These are not in any way helping your scenario, and are not providing restful sleep that heals the body during those hours spent in bed. Being able to rest in a light, relaxed state is highly beneficial to healing the body as well as resting the mind.[2]

It is important to understand that the restful body does drift between states of rest and sleep ranging from deep to light throughout the night. Sedated sleep is not healing, nor is it energizing sleep. This is information that you need to have for the purpose of recognizing your habits and determining how they affect the body, so you can manage your actions accordingly. Being aware of the kind of sleep you are getting is a huge step towards acquiring the sleep that you want.

I am not a sleep expert but I do know how crippling insomnia can be to a person's health. I am, however, a nutritional expert and I do know how food is metabolized in the body. What you eat all day will affect you how you sleep at night. Some foods are more obvious than others. People who won't drink coffee after two in the afternoon because they can't sleep know how this affects them. Consider this: The sugar substitutes that you consume all day are contributing to sleep quality. It is old news that sugar substitutes are potentially dangerous. Persistent inflammation may be causing your sleeplessness or poor sleep. If you are suffering with sinus infections and cannot breathe, or you are experiencing digestive unrest and cannot get comfortable, then the quality of your sleep will be poor.

I strongly recommend taking special care to investigate and discover what changes you can make to your daily health in order to ensure great healing sleep. Staying clear of food known or even suspected to keep a person awake is wise, especially while trying to uncover why your sleep is poor. Your diet may be the cause of persistent inflammation. Identifying the source of discomfort and healing that cause should be a restless sleeper's main priority. Great sleep leads to great health. The more rested a person is, the easier it will be to exercise and prepare for the day with good quality nutrition. This person will not need caffeine to keep them alert and can live in balance with their health.

A hyped-up, over-stimulated body will not sleep. This may be caused by too much sugary food or too much alcohol. It could be over-stimulated bacteria in the gut keeping you awake. Even too many probiotics can cause sleepless nights, since some kinds of bacteria are very active in the body, even when you rest. They are performing their own metabolic activities to stay alive. Too great a supply of certain bacteria can stem an imbalance within the gut. Imbalances are related to stress and a stressed situation stimulates activity. Sometimes what cures us in one way will harm us in other ways.

Take yogurt for example. The bacterial component of yogurt heals the gut and bolsters immune health, which is important in sleep. Calcium found in yogurt also helps sleep but too many active bacteria will keep some people awake at night. In addition to this, lactose is a sugar. Even in unsweetened yogurts that contain no added sugar, the natural sugars stimulate the body and may also keep someone awake. Keeping balance in how much you consume as well as the ingredients contained in what you consume in the evening (or before bed) is vital to successful sleep. This is why I encourage my clients not to eat after seven for a ten o'clock bedtime.

Inflammation caused by poor nutrition is the cause of almost every disease in the body, and is entirely avoidable. Good, restful, regular sleep patterns allow the body to recover and energize, like charging your phone. If the body has to be active in fighting inflammation caused by food, your rest may be poor. Choose food without added sweeteners and add your own natural ones instead. By controlling the amount of sweetener added to your food, you will significantly cut down on your sugar intake. Keeping control of your own sugar intake by simply adding your own sugar to food, rather than letting a food manufacturer do it, will give you control over how much you allow into your body. Natural sweeteners that are low in fructose and sucrose will digest more gently and will not result in blood sugar spikes that can keep a person awake.

I like to use organic sugar in my coffee, maple syrup in my food, and pure honey for almost everything else. Please note that all sugar raises blood sugar levels and is in no way recommended for diabetics. Try honey and maple syrup to substitute sugar in food, for maintaining an even blood sugar level. Pure honey is beneficial in many ways. Lessening the amount of sugar and sweetness in your food is preferable for everyone. A fatty liver, diabetes, obesity, sleeplessness, hyperactivity, poor concentration, mood disorders and skin breakouts are all on the short list of sugar-related health complications.

Regular exposure to super-sweet foods develops a hyper-sensitized palate for sweetness, meaning an individual will need very sweet things on the tongue in order to satisfy their craving for a sweet sensation. This is the equivalent of developing a tolerance and addiction to food or drinks. As this relates to good quality sleep, the sweeter your food is, the more food you will want in order to satisfy your cravings. The more you eat sweet food, the more the quality of your sleep declines. If a client is struggling with sleep, I focus a great deal on the sugar and sweet foods that they take in regularly. By taking control of their sugar intake, they often solve their sleep issues. Should they have restless children, we solve their sleep difficulties by limiting the sugar that they consume as well. I can directly link my clients' sleep success to the decrease or elimination of sugary foods and drinks in their diet. As their sleep improves, their health greatly improves.

As I shifted careers from interior designer to nutritional counselor, I wondered what the heck I had done all those years before. Did I waste my time? What could it all be for? It was all for this:

Make your bedroom a beautiful place.

I saw so many bedrooms as an interior designer and most were disasters. Many people figure no one will ever see inside their bedroom, so that must be the last place for design or decoration with beautiful things. Wrong! You deserve a beautiful and tranquil place to sleep. Make sure there is no clutter in your room, no chairs to hold piles of unfolded clothes (designate a neat place for your clothes like a hamper or the closet instead) and no boxes of files

31

that you have not gotten to organizing. Keep comfortable and simple bedding on your bed, just one or two blankets, and limit the amount of decorative pillows– they add clutter and offer more surfaces for dust mites, pollen and other allergens to cling to, especially since most decorative pillows are not machine washable. Find a bed that you can climb into easily for sleep and that can easily be made the next day. Do not keep a lot of electronics in your bedroom. Sleep experts recommend that you don't have a television in your room. I personally prefer no television but I realize that many people like to have a television in their bedrooms. If you must have a television in your room, set a timer and go to bed at bedtime.

I have a lovely client who was low on energy. She has a very long commute and a lot of responsibilities at work and at home. She once enjoyed being on social media in bed at night. The problem was that she was spending too much time late at night on her phone.

We set up a plan to set social medial boundaries. She is a very disciplined person and was eager to become motivated by the prospect of gaining more energy and better sleep. When she announced to her social world that she would turn off her devices at ten to go to sleep, she worried about their reactions. To her delight, there was tremendous support among her friends. She asked for help in keeping her goal to turn off socializing for better sleep and they all helped her do it. The best part was that she gained more sleep, woke well rested, was able to walk and exercise before work, and stopped smoking because she was too busy exercising to smoke. It was a win all the way around. After only one month, she lost weight and went from two packs a day to zero. Sleep became her main goal because, when she got good sleep, the rest of her life was well-managed and she could be at her best, making good choices rather than impulsive ones.

Please take a look at her success and realize that, when one area of your life is out of control, it will affect everything else. Understand that it is often the small changes that bring about huge successes.

Now that you know of the benefits of sleep, make sleep a priority. Make sleep in your bed without disruption your number one goal for tonight and successive nights. Let it become so essential to you that you find yourself longing for your new beautiful bedroom, without clutter and with soft, lovely, welcoming bedding to envelop your skin and nourish your health in the most passive way possible, while you are at rest.

Some great rituals to include in your bedtime:

Think about the ways that we prepare our babies for sleep. We bathe them, swaddle them, and tuck them in with stories. This nurturing ritual that you perform with your baby prepares them for much-needed rest. Preparing yourself for rest with a soothing ritual will do the same for you.

Always remove your street clothes before getting into bed. There are so many toxins from pesticides to filthy gunk from the street that attach to your clothes, and you don't want them on your bed sheets. Don't allow those street shoes into your bedroom. They were in public bathrooms and in wet muddy puddles; you don't want those toxic elements near your clean bed. Bathe the day's oils from your skin, hands and nails and change your clothes to comfortable pajamas. If you suffer from seasonal allergies, it is a great idea to shower and wash your hair in the evening. This is to clean off the pollen that gets stuck in your hair so as not to lie down and spend eight hours nose-to-pollen-infested-pillow.

I love to wash my face, use a bidet, and wash my feet before bed. I massage lavender-scented cream into my feet and hands, which relaxes me and prepares me for rest. The scent alone is part of the ritual of preparing for bed. I will actually sigh with comfortable relief as I slide into my fluffy clean bed, ready for sleep. I encourage you to find an effective ritual to include in your sleep-prep pattern. The preparation for rest is a trigger for the actual sleep itself. You not only deserve the beauty of sleep, your Health Beautiful self needs it.

Your Body is Built for Movement

The importance of exercise in a daily routine probably is not news to you. We are functional animals, built to move. I do extreme exercising and love every sweaty moment of it. I love my gym. It is a beautiful facility with more than its share of exercise classes and machines that I can utilize.

My husband loves to swim, but I stink at swimming. I can swim but I am a terrible swimmer for anything more than six laps, and even those laps are really bad. I hate it but I do it in the summer anyway.

I love jumping around and using weights and listening to very loud music. I love a very intense trainer who pushes me through the whole class. I love when I am next to a really fit person who works hard and keeps the energy up for me to tap into. One of my fitness instructors says I am relentless and so positive. This is true. I love those classes. Okay, this is not for everyone; I get it, just as swimming isn't for me. I tell you about what I love because I want to encourage you to find a physical activity that you love and incorporate it into your life.

For most people, limited time is what keeps them from exercise. I argue that we make time for the things that we want to do and maybe those people have not found their perfect activity just yet. My cousin Amy is a very busy woman. She found herself going to play pickup soccer in an adult league after working twelve-hour days. Why? She is very athletic, she loves sports, and she is a huge sports fan, going to games and watching games on television. She found a fitness activity that she also enjoys. Running on a treadmill will never get her to love exercise but playing soccer got her moving, even after long days. Added responsibilities and time constraints can be worked around. We make room for the activities that we want to do. Everyone knows that physical activity is essential to good health. Find what you enjoy with the understanding that your health benefits from daily physical movement.

Exercise through physical therapy is necessary after surgery and even during recovery from injuries. When I was attending college, I was a volunteer at the inpatient rehabilitation center at Metropolitan Hospital in New York City. I worked there for two years, aiding the physical therapists with patients in rehabilitation. The reasons for their hospitalization included disease, gunshot wounds, head trauma, stroke, and scaffolding accidents. Many had severe brain and spinal cord injuries. Our responsibilities included exercising along with patients as they regained movement in their limbs and the ability to function. The sheer determination of some patients as they worked through their debilitating injuries and came back to full function was incredibly moving and truly inspirational. Many of these patients were completely immobile and unable to move their limbs when we started their physical therapy. Many came through significant odds and made incredible leaps to be close to fully functioning.

I will always remember one man, Mr. Williams, who had fallen from scaffolding. When I met him, he could not move a single muscle because he had a partially severed spinal cord. He worked so hard at his recovery. He made every effort, with sweat and tears, trying to make his muscles move. By the time the semester ended and my hours were done, I was throwing him a fifteen pound medicine ball and he was catching it while seated, then throwing it back to me. That is willpower and unwavering determination. That is confidence and inspiration.

Sometimes, when I hear of someone who complains that they don't want to exercise, I think of Mr. Williams and Tony, another patient who was a gunshot victim. He was living with significant pain, yet he would still get on the basketball court in his wheelchair to play. I think about how nothing could stand between them and their bodies' needs to move and be active. We all have a personal challenge that may interfere with our exercise routine. Taking a look at the human body and how it needs to exercise may help to motivate you past any excuses you may have.

I know many women and men who love to play tennis and golf, and many more who will kayak or coach basketball for their kids. Sports are well honored and the benefits of playing sports are understood by many. And yet, I see dads who can't run across the field where they coach twenty kids in lacrosse. They obviously love the sport but they are in desperate need of exercise. I say, join a league and play yourself.

A treadmill is easy to use and offers a time and mile measurement for those who want to gauge their exercise in that way. Taking a class or joining a team is so much more fun. The social aspect of exercise helps to keep people involved in their routines. No one has to join an Iron Man event to prove that they can do it, although some might respond to a huge, challenging goal as motivation to exercise. As in nutrition, everyone has different needs. Meeting those needs will keep you in great physical health.

It is not a good idea to allow age to stop you from moving. This bad habit is starting at younger and younger ages. My husband's grandmother just passed away at age ninety-three. She was only sick for a very short time and passed quickly and peacefully. She was very strong and died an independent woman. She tended her own garden and exercised daily for all of her life. At age sixty-four, she picked up cross-country skiing. She swam in the cold lakes of Germany all throughout her life. She practiced tai chi and made physical activity a huge priority in her life. I have immense respect for her and we will miss her inspirational phone calls and visits very much.

I challenge you to be the person who can walk upright into their doctor's office and leave without any new prescriptions. Leave your checkups with total confidence and the understanding that you are an example of great health. Let your medical personnel tell you that you are the picture of health. This is a real goal for me. It is achievable for anyone who wants it. You need to make the decision to love yourself and love your life enough to live it with vitality and longevity, not in a medicated state filled with glucose strips and antibiotics. So many people expect illness to be a part of life, especially as they age. It is a shame to accept such a fate. I prefer to live with the expectation of surprise, love, and adventure, not endless visits to the doctor and time spent waiting for results. You can do this, you just need to want it badly enough.

Go for it. Find that yoga or Zumba class; find that dance jam or tennis team; go for long hikes or bike rides. There is something out there for anyone who wants to keep fit and strong.

The potential benefits of exercise are tremendous. One perfect example is balance. A friend that I exercise with recently told me about a scene that she witnessed while waiting for her train to New York City. A man of about sixty-five lost his footing on a train platform and fell onto the tracks as the train was approaching. Several other people had to jump in and pull him to safety. The man was terrified, as he should have been; it was an awful experience. What I took away from this story is that I need to be able to catch myself before I fall, and to have the strength to be able to lift my own body out of a hole if I'm ever required to do so. Even if you don't play sports or exercise a lot, you should at least be able to hold yourself in a balanced position on one foot, and be able to get yourself up and out of danger.

I understand that I sound tough but I truly care about everyone's health. I want people to know how great it feels to be able to carry your own weight and move your own body in any position you need to be in. Physical activity improves your body from head to toe. There are cognitive benefits to engaging in exercise activities that are strenuous while concentrating on moving your body in specific ways, i.e. aerobics, basketball or tennis. This kind of activity is especially beneficial for maintaining cognitive longevity. It causes all of your systems to be activated in a controlled and intentional way. Strive to achieve great balance, strength, cardiovascular endurance, and flexibility as a part of your healthy living plan for a long and happy life.

I encourage you to get a friend to accompany you or to join a fitness studio where you may make friends. Adding a social element to your physical activities will keep you going back and will help you to enjoy the time spent doing that activity. Whether it is a team sport or an individual practice, making connections with other people who do the same type of exercise is helpful for both motivation and for inspiration. People who are extremely athletic enjoy motivating others. Before classes, my gym friends and I all chat and laugh. We look forward to seeing each other and celebrate each other's accomplishments after class. Team members engage in celebrations and laughter while playing their team sports, and it is always more fun to run outside with your kids or dog than it is to stay locked away at your desk. Find a way to incorporate exercise into your Health Beautiful life. It will bring you and your circle of friends closer to each other and happier in your long, lovely lives.

A Good Shvitz

In many cultures around the world, sweating is a bonding and healing rite of passage. I heard a story told by a New York author on the MOTH radio hour. The speaker described his Jewish grandfather and father who would go to steam rooms together, to groan or grunt in a ceremonial sigh of toxin release and to experience the bonding between men of a certain age and level of wisdom. He had wanted to achieve this bond himself and to become a part of this ceremony for a long time. It was a very funny story but the point was not lost. Sweating in a ceremonial steam room to detoxify the liver and the skin is not just a tradition, but an extremely healing ritual as well.

Try to incorporate sweating into a daily practice, either in a sauna or through exercise. Exertion that triggers a sweating response is normal and healthy. There is a natural cooling down and regulatory response that occurs in all human beings. This is basic biology. Sweating is the body's attempt to regulate temperature and release toxins. Exercise is recommended by every medical and health professional. If you are not exercising because you do not like to sweat, know that the more your body learns to anticipate the exertion and exercise, the more likely it is to generate a clean sweat as a healthy response. I know that for some the feeling of being sweaty is uncomfortable, but keep in mind that a daily sweat will clean out toxins that can suppress immune response.

I recommend that you exercise or steam daily, or at least several times a week if that is not feasible. If you have access to a sauna, I highly recommend using it for a dry sweat, as this is the preferred way to detox. Again, try to ritualize the practice. Just as you might light a candle at a dinner party or send emails at a certain time each day, incorporate a sweating detox into your lifestyle as a step toward healthy immunity and a good, clean body inside and out.

Those who cannot sweat easily may be suffering from a thyroid imbalance, as may those who sweat a lot without much exertion. I attended a "clean liver" seminar in New York City, hosted by Dr. Peter Bongiorno ND, LAc, where he spoke about his patients, many of whom had done a "cleanse" with powdered drinks in an effort to lose weight or cleanse their bodies of toxins. He described the scenario, where the constant passing of liquid through their intestinal tracts sometimes causes a block in the intestinal release of bowel movements and reintroduces those toxins back into the body. Peristalsis is the natural wavelike movement that moves your food all the way through your digestive tract. Stimulating peristalsis with drinks or juicing too much will slow the metabolic absorption of nutrients. There are specific chemicals in the intestinal tract that create the exact consistency and makeup for perfect absorption of nutrients. The backup of bowel release and slowing of peristalsis may be toxic, and the liver may be sending the very toxins that the cleanse was supposed to release right back into the body. Dr. Bongiorno and I recommend real, whole, natural dietary fiber in the form of vegetables along with water to cleanse the body of toxins.

Let water and dietary fiber found in vegetables cause good bowel movements and add a sweat to pour out the toxins from the largest organ– your skin. Eventually, as the intestinal tract and the heat-regulating systems in the body normalize, you will sweat less while just hanging around, and sweat more when exercising. This is a normal response to cardio encouragement. Standing still and sweating is not a good response to normal temperatures. Obviously, high temperatures during hot days will cause you to sweat in order to cool you down, but if you cannot regulate the sweat or cool down easily, understand that your built-in regulatory system has been disrupted. This could be the result of toxin-saturated organs. Pure food and intentional sweating may heal this reaction.

Honor Thy Food

Food is a necessary part of life, but lots of social norms and cultural expectations dictate our relationships with food. Children depend on their parents to feed them and keep them alive and well. Adults use food to celebrate and reward themselves and others. They like to shower children with sweet foods to let them know that they are loved. Adolescents sometimes try to control their own lives with food through deprivation or indulgence. Women often feel guilty about eating food, referring to being "good" by eating small quantities of food or being "bad" by eating fat-rich food. Men feel social pressure about not restricting their food intake. They are bombarded with these messages and encouraged to eat large amounts of bar food, or "masculine" food.

Feeling pulled in conflicting directions while trying to serve yourself and your family with nourishment can be overwhelming. Often, my clients will discuss the uncomfortable feelings they have when they are trying to make changes to their food routine. They don't want to be the difficult one, rejecting restaurant suggestions made by friends who want a night out, or saying no to their family member that wants to order in rather than cook together. They don't want to appear too health conscious because they don't want to come across as a health nut. They offer bowls of chips or order pizza when their children have friends over because they want the kids to feel they were treated well during their stay. I can't count how many people have told me that they feel bad giving their family vegetables instead of meatballs.

These are mostly self-imposed emotions that clients use as excuses to keep them from reaching their own goals. As we reveal the underlying reasons for these emotions, they soon discover that their friends want to eat out at healthy places too, and their kids' friends will eat anything that they offer, even a vegetable platter. Their spouse enjoys home cooking when they make it simple and ritualize the process with music and laughter. It turns out that so much of what keeps us in harmful routines are negative conversations that we are having in our own heads. They are often our own projection of what we think of ourselves, not what is actually happening.

Take the example of my clients in the corporate environment where we implemented a no-sweets break room. One strategy that people practiced is when it came time to order lunch was this: one person would usually speak up and offer the suggestion of ordering healthy choices for lunch. They never were rejected because the power of their healthy lunch suggestion was strong, and spoken with confidence. Everyone loved being able to eat and stay on their own course toward health.

Healthy meals and healthy celebrations with food are contagious. People feel honored when someone goes the extra mile to make sure that the food they celebrate with is healthy and good to eat. Takeout pizza is not much of a celebration. Think about how you honor celebrations with food and examine what is holding you in a rut, then make a change. It will be appreciated.

The food industry relies on the emotional effect that food has on people in order to sell them *more* food. There is no question that food taps into human emotion. I encourage you and your family members to rethink and restructure your relationship with food. Food sustains us, and we celebrate and honor our accomplishments with it. It makes us feel good when we are sick and makes us feel satisfied when we are hungry. Honor yourself, your celebrations and your life with the highest quality food that you can get. Let your new mantra be: "No junk for me, not now, not ever again." Your new relationship with food will honor and respect the power that it possesses over you. Place it in a clean place and serve it with a sense of ritual and love.

Once you respect the ways in which food sustains your life and how good food choices make you feel, your relationship with food becomes more positive. You will find yourself feeling proud of your choices and respectful of the positive reactions that friends and family have toward you and the delicious culinary experiences that you expose them to. Experiencing new healthy restaurants and delicious meals that you learned to make from healthy cookbooks is exciting. You will begin to enjoy how much easier your life is without feeling sick or tired after eating a meal. A positive relationship with a necessity like food will lead to nutritional, emotional and overall success in all aspects of life. As you learn to prepare and use food as fuel each day, your daily accomplishments are more easily met.

A positive relationship with food will increase your energy and confidence in yourself. You will become more focused and will gain the ability to pause easily when you need a break because your focus has shifted toward supporting your health. Instead of breaking up your workday to go to the lunchroom for cake or donuts, you may choose to go for a walk instead. Your newfound confidence in your health will put you on a path that is unwavering. The excuses that kept you sick and tired all the time become a threat to this newfound feeling of exhilarating health, so you dare not use them again. The time that you take to shop in new places and make your own meals cannot compare to the sluggishness you once felt and the trips to pharmacies and doctors that your unhealthy self once demanded. The ease with which you accomplish your work becomes so encouraging that you will actually look forward to working and finishing each task.

As you begin to select food that doesn't result in hormone fluctuations or the ups and downs of your blood sugar levels, your attitude towards people and relationships becomes more balanced. We have all experienced the short fuse of someone who is irritable because of a blood sugar drop and may even have been the one who was irritated at others.

Respecting the power that food has to support your nutritional needs develops a cognitive relationship, rather than an emotional relationship, to your food selections. The relationship that you have with food becomes more loving because the result of your food choices is making you feel great. This feeling of love toward yourself is expressed with each meal and each decision that you make to feed your body with great nutritious food. Being healthy will bring the rest of your world together. The feeling of accomplishing something amazing and meeting your responsibilities with greatness is all made easier when you are healthy. Taking control of your health is the way to gain control of your life. This is in your power. It's so incredibly rewarding.

Beautiful Pantry, Beautiful Cooking, Beautiful Life

The place where you keep your food should be clean and free of clutter. When I was an interior designer, I entered many kitchens and was baffled by the overstocked cabinets and overflowing drawers. Even before I moved into nutrition, I could see a correlation between the clutter and unhealthy foods in a kitchen, and the sickly appearance of the homeowner. It is easy to de-clutter your kitchen without going through a complete $60,000 kitchen renovation. There are some simple steps in organizing and stocking your cabinets with health-promoting necessities as you free yourself from junk foods and treat yourself with health foods.

Take a look at a grocery store like Whole Foods, whose shoppers are often very conscientious about all aspects of their food selection. The Whole Foods shopper looks for organic, pasture-raised, grass-fed, hormone- and antibiotic-free, local, sustainable and healthy food. The shelves are clean and the packaging is simple. The produce is well stocked but not excessively so; you won't find huge displays with towering pyramids of food. There is a reason for this. Clean, simple appearances in a supermarket convey clean, uncomplicated lives. Who doesn't want that? I encourage you to do the following in your kitchen.

7 Remove any food products that have an ingredient list longer than 7 items.

For the heavyweights ready to dive into ultra-clean living, remove the items that contain more than 3 ingredients. These could be items such as taco seasoning mix or salad dressing in a bottle, mayonnaise and cereal bars. The meals that you make will contain more than 7 ingredients, but each added ingredient is just 1 item added, not 12. For example, when I make chili I add a lot of individual ingredients that are all selected with care: dried chili peppers (1 ingredient), onions (1), tomatoes (1), and so on. If I were to add a package of chili seasoning mix it would be chili mix (16 ingredients in the powdered mix), canned tomatoes (3), onion (1), and so on.

The idea is to eliminate unnecessary chemicals and processed ingredients that you use regularly from your daily eating routine. By conducting this exercise and cleaning out your pantry, you will remove harmful, highly processed, and usually shockingly hidden ingredients from your diet. Cleaning the pantry first will clean up your cooking and clean up your health. This is an empowering and thoroughly educational exercise.

A long ingredient list is an indicator of highly processed food. For instance, the peanut butter that I purchase has an ingredient list with two items: *organic peanuts and sea salt.* That is all. If you read the ingredients on many popular mainstream jars of peanut butter, you typically will see a much longer list. Many items are red flags for artificial chemicals that may cause a variety of health complications. I can rattle off a list of exactly what I eat in a day, down to the individual ingredients. If you are eating food that has a long list of ingredients, you will never be clean and free from chemicals in your body. Keep your food uncomplicated and you will keep your life simple. See Appendix B (p. 142) for an actual ingredient list from a popular food product.

The biochemical reactions that take place while digesting

and absorbing food are corrupted by the unusable chemical compounds found in processed food. There are many studies that indicate that the endocrine system is significantly disrupted by chemicals and products ingested with food.[3] Such disruptions can range from polycystic ovary disease to autoimmune disease. These same studies find that, by simply removing the processed foods and even avoiding certain containers that hold food–like cans and plastic containers–from a patient's diet, blood levels normalized within as little as three days.

That is a powerful result, first because it shows that for certain people the simple addition of chemicals in food and certain containers that hold food results in disruption of one of their regulatory systems, but also because the body is so incredibly efficient that it is able to clean and release the foreign bodies within only three days. That is remarkable. These results are encouraging and they show that the human body is capable of healing itself on its own when given a chance.

I love the human body– it is amazing to me. Even if you don't suffer from severe health complications such as autoimmune disease, you may be suffering from chronic infections, inflammation, skin irritation, sleeplessness or excess weight. While many people may find temporary relief with medication, that only puts a band-aid on illnesses that compound when ignored. Solving the main cause of such illnesses will give you a lifetime of relief, while that provided by medication may only last for four to six hours.

Side Rant: Don't even get me started on the side effects of medication. The physical complications can't even be listed on the bottle. You have to go online to see the long list of side effects, almost all of which include the warning that in rare instances it may cause death: *warning, may cause death...*

2 Eliminate all food that contains corn syrup and corn byproducts.

Corn syrup is a major ingredient in very poor quality foods. It is used for added flavor, as a filler or preservative, and to create a less expensive product for the manufacturer. None of these uses support your health. High fructose corn syrup (HFCS) and other modified corn products have been shown to contribute to the onset of several serious diseases. HFCS creates a super-sweet flavor and a significant spike in blood sugar. Indigestible in the body, it can lead to fatty liver disease. Fatty liver is often a prelude to significant complex diseases.[4] It is a diet-related disease and diet-altering solutions are recommended.[5]

The effects of added sugar have been well documented in children. Sugary foods like soda and cereal can wreak havoc in their bodies, affecting their organs, blood and brains. Small children may become irritable, difficult and hyper when given sugary food. You can see this in action when a kid is given candy and five minutes later they are jumping around and running in circles. Imagine having to sit still in class with these types of foods in your system.

A number of behavioral challenges seen in elementary schools could be solved with the removal of sugar-enhanced food, most of which is low in dietary fiber and highly processed. Looking at the ingredient list is the key to detecting these products. A rule of thumb is, if you cannot identify the ingredient then don't eat it, and for goodness sake don't give it to your kids. I mention this because there are many phrasings for corn products on food labels that may not be perfectly clear. Using this guideline, you will want to bring home food that comes from easily identified sources. To be perfectly clear:

- Anything ending in –ose is a sugar.
- If you don't recognize and are unable to pinpoint the original source of an ingredient, don't include it in your diet.

Anything described as a corn product in the ingredient list is a sugar-based preservative, enhancer or filler. Corn farming today is a major industry that relies on genetically modified plants, pesticides, herbicides and the use of heavy-duty chemical fertilizers, resulting in a product I do not wish to feed my family. By staying away from food with added corn products, we are able to avoid one major source of potentially harmful foods. For corn on the cob we choose local and organic corn while in season, and we pop organic popcorn in an air popper, then add our own toppings (which my thirteen-year-old's friends beg for when they come over). We always select organic whole kernel corn and never include corn flour in anything that we eat. I highly recommend this as a guideline for you, in order to keep harmful chemicals and added sugar out of your diet.

Excess weight is generally the result of a diet associated with excessive sugar and sugary foods like juice and sports drinks. Excess fat is linked to many health complications. The potential detrimental effects of being overweight and addicted to sugar are overwhelming, especially for children and adolescents. The CDC lists the serious and complex social and health difficulties and diseases acquired by obese children.[6] Young children have difficulty playing and being active. They can also be too active. This often results in disciplinary action followed by retreat that's combined with brain fog after the sugar wears off, which isolates them.

The heightened sweetness in foods with added sugar and sugar substitutes that many children are given regularly lay the ground work for detesting natural real food.[7] This complicates a parent's job when trying to give vegetables and unsweetened food to their kids, resulting in a terrible cycle of tantrums and emotional mood swings. I hear from many clients about how their kids won't eat anything. I encourage them to try to feed the kids absolutely no products with added sugar in the effort to wean their kids from sugar addiction. As is the case with withdrawal from any drug, it will take a tremendous effort of will and support.

This is not to say all sweet products should be eliminated, only those containing unnecessary added sugar. Refusing candy but adding your own honey to homemade oatmeal is fine, because you have control over how much is added. At my house we use pure maple syrup, which contains low levels of fructose. Homemade or plain yogurt with honey or maple syrup is good, whereas store bought selections that are colored, flavored and low-calorie are not. The added sugar is usually found in much higher quantities than you would add to your own yogurt and the added coloring or artificial ingredients support obesity, not excellent health.

A significant part of my nutritional counseling program with families deals with weaning the kids from processed foods and excessive amounts of sugar in their diets as they achieve success in their health. There is a significant addiction in this country to sugar. It is out of control. The brain likes sugar because sugar found in fruit means energy for the brain. Before there were grocery stores, when humans had to gather their energy from natural sources like fruit, we developed "good" messages from the brain to eat this sweet fruit to continue giving the body quick reliable energy. Unfortunately, the brain messaging has stayed even though the source of sugar has been significantly altered. The amount of sugar eaten today is significantly more than humans need for survival. Even though we are constantly reminded by health and wellness professionals to stop, slow down and remove sugar, we still go to it even though it is killing us.

The addiction to these instinctive forces that drive us to desire and eat sugar almost cripples some of my clients. Being drawn to something that they know is dangerous and making them miserable is confusing and frustrating. This is why we work at removing all sugar that is added to their food by anyone other than themselves– a successful strategy for beating sugar addiction. As long as they are letting food manufacturers add the sugar to their food, they are removed from the action and the addiction is not related clearly to their own action. They see a food like cereal and think breakfast. By simply reading the ingredients and understanding that corn byproducts mean sugar to their bodies, they realize that it is the same as pouring a bowl of sugar for breakfast. Making the connection to your food is a key part in understanding what it is that you are actually eating. The cleaning out of corn products and sugary food from your pantry is essential to overall health, especially for those with sugar addiction.

Considering the constant brain fog (that unfocused and tired feeling that comes with sleeplessness, sugar drops, starvation and too much stress) that many of us experience in our lives, it is obvious why some brains are excited by sweet tastes. As a protective act for your future health and the health of your entire family, I urge you to cleanse your pantry of sugar. By eliminating all products that contain added sugar, you are ten steps ahead of the game.

Making your pantry free from added corn products will likely clean out a junk food junkie's entire kitchen. This process will shock you when you do it at your home. Corn syrup and corn byproducts are found in the most likely *and* unlikely of places.

3 Eliminate food that is older than 1 month.

While you are at it, get rid of those rotting, soggy or limp vegetables that dwell at the back of the refrigerator. Properly stored items that have a longer shelf life will be kept fresh, like dried goods and foods that do not spoil quickly such as vinegar. Oil-based foods like nut spreads and nuts as well as all oils go rancid, so keeping a close eye on this will make your food taste better. Condiments bought in amounts that suit your demands will rotate out at a healthy pace; a huge container of mustard is unnecessary for someone who uses it 2 times a month. Consider the cost compared to the use and how you plan to store your food. If an item is taking up a lot of space in a pantry or refrigerator that has limited space, it will be a burden. The plan to get healthy has a lot to do with removing burdens from your life.

So put on those rubber gloves and get to it. Toss all those old, limp carrots at the bottom of the vegetable crisper drawer, and any old onion skins floating around the refrigerator. Get that old frozen tomato sauce from two years ago out of the freezer and into the garbage.

Why don't you want old food in your refrigerator? Because you are not eating old food anymore. Not only is it potentially dangerous, it's really undesirable. I have explained that the purpose of this book is to lead you towards eating the highest quality food that you can get. At the very least, you shouldn't have to eat old food.

What does this mean for your health? The food that we eat is there to provide energy so that we can function. Every single client that I have ever encountered has wanted more energy, among other goals. Eating fresh food is a perfect way to acquire as much energy as you can with each meal. Freshly purchased local produce in your refrigerator is highly desirable. Everyone prefers a fresh, crisp and brightly colored vegetable over a soggy old one. This may be an acquired taste for some, especially for those who never experienced fresh items growing up, either due to income or location.

Then there is this one little problem... warehouse-style big box store shopping. Yikes! Here is a streamlined version of my argument. Like it or not, you can simplify your life by giving up shopping in bulk.

- The big box stores take time and energy from your life.
- It is extremely costly to shop there.
- The packaging is difficult to handle.
- The unpacking and repacking of meat, vegetables, dairy products and dried goods is overwhelming.
- The food is sold in quantities that are too large and thus it spoils, creating excess waste and wasted money!

Plan to shop at a few markets, and shop often. You need the basics on hand regularly but you do not need a ½ gallon tub of cream cheese. The day we liberated ourselves from the big box store was a good day for my family.

- First, we saved hundreds of dollars each month by not going to big box stores.
- Second, we eliminated the hassle of navigating the huge oversized lot with oversized cars and oversized carts, searching for a spot to park.
- Third, we eliminated the time-consuming hassle of going through enormous warehouses with too many people to get only some of our groceries.
- Fourth, the backbreaking lugging of giant bulky boxes into and out of our carts, then into and out of our car, then into the house was no longer my problem.
- Fifth, I do not have to repackage large quantities of food and organize my freezer, then remember to thaw and use the food that is meant to last a week and make it last five weeks instead by keeping track of what I bought and when it was bought. This was an overwhelming process and much of the stored food was usually thrown away.
- Sixth, I no longer had to wait on long return lines to get money back for food that, once I got home and opened the large package, turned out to be moldy or spoiled (this happened every single time without fail, especially with prepackaged produce).
- Finally, arguments no longer ensue over who has to do all of the abovementioned tasks. My dear friend who won't give up her big box store literally takes one entire day to shop, and it costs her $400-500 dollars each time. Does spending that much really make it worth saving a couple dollars on razors? I don't think so.

Make a plan for your meals starting at the beginning of the week. Anticipate what you are planning to eat on Thursday and prep for it while cooking Monday's dinner. For example, while roasting sweet potatoes, also roast other vegetables for another dinner. Depending on the season, I go to various places for food. The reason is that I want my vegetables to have been harvested as close as possible to the time that I eat them. Have criteria for selecting the food that you buy. Being from Long Island, it is easy for me to think of all of my food in the same way that I select fish: fresh, clean, and from somewhere that I trust. The same holds true for the rest of your food. Try to keep these criteria for your kitchen, your food, and your body. Knowing how fresh the food is will encourage you to eat it quickly and enjoy the benefits.

4 Minimize your pantry items and cookware.

It is not necessary to have four spatulas and six ladles and fifteen knives on hand at all times. I hear from every overwhelmed cook that they don't have the space to cook, or they can't bring themselves to enjoy cooking. I point out that they likely have too many options. Limit your cookware to regularly used tools and appliances. Jerry Seinfeld recently did a stand-up bit about why people need to get rid of their useless garbage. He jokes about when people bring a new gadget into the house. You place it on your dining room table and unwrap it with excitement, then you place it in a cabinet in the kitchen. After a few weeks, you move it into a closet and eventually it ends up in the garage. Before you know it, you're trying to sell it on eBay.[8] Does that sound familiar? The point is to only buy items that you will use regularly, and keep it simple. Simplify your kitchen and your cooking will follow. Spend your time wisely in the kitchen without fussy utensils and clutter so that the cooking experience is easy and positive.

5 Place perishable food up front in your refrigerator and cabinets and keep a steady rotation of dry goods and condiments, like mustard and hot sauces.

You don't want to keep old food around. The energy and flavor of the food is depleted, and who wants to eat food without energy or flavor?

While you are at it, rotate out your travel cup collection and your mismatched plates and glasses as well. Eating on pretty dishes is an important part of living beautifully. When you eat mindfully and honor your food by serving it on a beautiful plate, and settle down to a clean and lovely table, you digest better, the food tastes better, and most importantly, you are giving priority to your food and thus to your body.

6 Keep the kitchen free of non-kitchen items.

Computers, electronic tablets, coupons and secretarial items like office supplies and mail and junk drawers do not belong in the kitchen. Consider this: food is the sustenance that keeps you alive. Junk, clutter, and negative distractions have no place in the space where you cook and eat your meals. Use your drawers to lay out your cooking utensils for easy access, and put your herbs, salt and olive oil in beautiful containers on the countertop. Keep a clean cutting board on the counter and reserve it for cooking purposes only. The cooking experience in a beautiful kitchen that facilitates easy access to useful tools is a delightful one. A positive, well-planned environment may entice you to cook your meals at home. Cooking your beautiful food in a beautiful environment is an essential part of your Health Beautiful lifestyle.

Fire Your Diet

Diets don't work because they are often restrictive and negative. Going on a diet suggests it will come to an end. The diet is a dreaded time filled with hunger, crankiness, struggle and frustration. Weighing oneself daily gives you an exact number to hate yourself with all day long. A traditional diet frequently consists of measuring and counting, guilt over cheating, eating less on Fridays because you want to drink more and then working extra hard on Saturdays to make up for it all. It is utterly hopeless, this dieting stuff.

The conversation around diets is always about *giving up*. If you give up this food, you will lose weight and be a winner. But winners never give up, only quitters and losers give up. So what is the message? Is it that we need to be quitters in order to win? Wow, so much judgment is attached to all that winning and losing and quitting and giving up. No wonder people are frustrated with their diets. The message in itself is distracting and completely contradictory. Instinctively, we know this. Everyone who has been on a diet and then goes on another diet knows the truth: Diets don't work, not for your life and not for your health.

A diet is something that people go on and off of, gaining and losing, then gaining again. In reality, starvation and deprivation is the worst way to gain anything, especially in terms of your health.

The diet industry makes millions by selling various products. They sell you things like 100-calorie snacks. The idea is that by eating a bag of 100-calorie cookies you will become skinny, which is ridiculous. Eating cookies may raise sugar levels and blood pressure, and may cause weight gain, even a 100-calorie bag. Many people struggle with cravings that are temporarily satisfied by cookies. I encourage my clients to enjoy something sweet each day. Not an entire box of cookies but something special and sweet. The reason that they are craving this sweet in the first place may be far beyond the nutritional elements of food and may more specifically be about a deeper desire for love. A 100-calorie snack bag will never satisfy those desires.

The way to end dieting forever is to understand your struggle between food and satisfaction, and to deliver your body what it needs, not what you think you want. The body will cross messages and create a craving for candy because you are running low on energy. What you need is to recharge, and sleep would be the best solution. This is often the cross-messaging that goes on with nighttime snacking. You crave something to eat late at night because the body is out of energy at the end of the day. Simply going to sleep rather than going to the refrigerator could resolve your craving and support your health.

A younger client who craved a boy's kiss would eat two chocolate Hershey's Kisses each night right before bed. She did what she could to satisfy that desire. Eating chocolate at 11:30 at night, she appeared to have an inability to control her late-night snacking. Through exploring the parts of her life that were out of balance, we uncovered her desire for a boy's love. Once she understood what was happening, she became conscious of her actions in a whole new way. We were able to create strategies to cope with her needs in healthy ways. The balance that she struck in this aspect of her life created a ripple effect, with positive results throughout.

Late-night snacking can make people feel disappointed with themselves. As we begin our journey together, my clients often talk to me about how they struggle all day with dieting and blow it at night, seemingly without control of themselves. Becoming liberated from this negative association with food and fostering impulse control are strategies that we work on together. It takes honest, introspective sessions.

Many of my clients gain control of their lives as they are released from the pull of unhealthy habits and work to create supportive new habits. Once they build a healthy relationship with snacking and impulses, other healthy relationships become a part of their lives. People in loveless marriages often crave super-sugary foods, so sometimes craving something sweet is actually a misinterpretation of a craving for an emotional connection that is lacking in their personal relationships. It is my job as a nutritional counselor to listen to clients and help them to figure out what drives cravings. It is also my job to recommend healthy solutions that are specific to the needs of my clients.

Nutritional counseling reaches far beyond food selection. The intense dialog and investigation of where people have balance and where they lack balance in their lives is exactly what I do. My clients are on a quest to be Health Beautiful. Whether we meet in person or conduct our sessions over the phone or Skype, I listen carefully, drawing on strengths that create fulfillment in one area of life and helping to use those strengths to strike a similar balance in areas that need improvement. Our sessions involve listening and strategizing, along with creating good eating habits and developing nutritional support, thus allowing my clients to gain control in all aspects of their lives.

A diet never feels good

The dieting process is filled with deprivation and restriction. People tend to restrict their calories in an attempt to lose weight. They may gain some control over portion size and this may be a good thing, but they are often misguided by calorie counts. A calorie-restricted diet leaves nutrition out of the picture. By restricting calories, you can still be overweight and dissatisfied with your health.

Eating a bag of low-calorie cookies on your diet is using calories as your guide to weight loss. It may qualify as an acceptable choice on some diet plans, but it is actually a poor addition to your body that deprives it of nutrition. The problem is that a cookie is a cookie, and no matter the calorie count, it is not aiding your weight loss success. It is an industry trick and an advertising gimmick to appeal to your weakness for sweet foods, which seduces you with a promise of low calorie count into buying their product.

There is a great deal of research done by the marketing departments of food companies to discover new ways to get people to commit to buying products. Sugary milk chocolate is highly addictive, even in a low-calorie baggie. Big food companies rely on your impulses, coupled with your carefully-cultivated sugar addiction, to keep you committed to the calorie game and keep them in business. A diet that uses restriction and a white-knuckle approach to weight loss is a losing battle. You lose your commitment and you lose self-motivation. The only thing you cannot count on losing for good is weight.

Side Rant: Sugar is highly addictive, especially when it comes in the form of snack-sized baggies of pulverized, artificial chemical-ridden and industrialized snacks. Those 100-calorie snacks are like little baggies of drugs that can be sold legally in stores. The supermarket supplies these baggies of drugs readily to their customers. The manufacturers label the front of the packages with words like honest, fat free, sugar free, gluten free, organic, only one point, and so on. The truth is that you will never be a healthy weight if you are eating snack bags of food. Don't believe the nonsense. The ad industry relies on your weakness and vulnerability to impulse-driven purchases, so they want you to believe in their product and buy more. The calorie restriction is supposed to somehow work miracles on your hips and tomorrow you will slide right into those size four skinny jeans and run off to marry the most wonderful man in the world. Nope, not true.

You are better than a 100-calorie baggie of sugar, salt, and pulverized flour that is injected with chemicals to adhere the gooey center to the dusty "cookie" crust. You deserve the best and this book is meant to teach you about how to feed yourself, to nourish your cells into becoming perfect machines with perfect metabolizing ability.

My gift to you is a new mindset: I am eating my way to a perfect body and beautiful health. I will never diet, never ever again!

I Love You, so I'm Telling You

Protein powders don't make you skinny, and they do not proclaim to make you skinny on the package. It is actually illegal for manufacturers to make this claim since it cannot be scientifically proven, yet every day trainers will recommend protein powders to their clients for weight loss. Your body needs nutrition and has the ability to break down, interpret, and absorb nutrients naturally. Suggesting that using a protein powder to accomplish this also suggests that the body is incapable of doing its job, which is shameful. Your body is a perfect machine with ideal mechanics whose specific purpose is to keep you in perfect health. Here are the facts about protein powders and other processed powders that some people add to their drinks in place of real, natural, whole food.

The truth

The facts

The reality is...

- If you are fat, you are eating crap.

It's that simple.

- Diets are unnecessary.
- Powders are unnecessary.
- Struggling with 30-day detox and weight loss challenges is unnecessary.
- If you want to be thin, you have to quit eating nonfood items.

I can't say it often enough, so here it is again: The cell is designed perfectly. It will read the nutritional information you give it to read. When you give it pizza to read, it will see sugar and melted fat that's probably combined with processed meat filled with chemicals. I'm not saying that you can't eat pizza; I'm saying that when you do eat pizza, you are giving nothing of value to the body. No nutrients, no vitamins, no usable fat, no usable proteins. You are not supplying your body with antioxidants or dietary fiber. When you feed the cells pizza, you give nothing of nutritional value, and therefore the body thinks it is starving.

The reason for this is that the body can only live on nutritional information, and the specific information that it needs is comprised of vitamins, minerals, antioxidants, fiber, fats, carbohydrates and so on. But the body is also designed to break down and read the food with its built-in mechanisms. When the body is given protein powders, the breaking down of the food is eliminated and thus bypassed for immediate intestinal absorption. Specific bonds that are created through chewing whole natural food do not occur with protein powder drinks and juiced vegetables and fruits.

The bonds that are made during digestion are perfect for the villi in the intestines to read and pass on to be used in the body. The use of a protein powder for rapid absorption of these nutrients leaves many steps out of your natural digestive process. This is part of the reason why people may develop a bloated belly on protein powders and prolonged juice diet regimens. The other reason is that a message of low nutrients is relayed to the regulatory system. As a result, alarms in the body are triggered for a state of malnutrition. Some initial weight loss may occur, but that will subside and subsequently reverse. This is because the main reason for the weight gain was never addressed in the first place. Coupled with dietary restriction and skipping meals, plus bypassing the digestive process, the body unravels into a total metabolic shutdown.

The digestive system takes up the majority of the human

body. It includes the digestive tract and affects every drop of blood in your body. You ARE what you EAT. Eating non-nutritious food, rushing the process or bypassing the steps of feeding the body nutritious information, is foolish if you are hoping to gain or maintain great health. Eating real, natural, whole food is the only way to safely and successfully create perfect balance in your body. This is the only quick fix in becoming healthy.

You do not need powdered vitamins when you are preparing a perfect meal. Your body knows exactly how to decode and take in information that makes every inch of your body perfect. Health Beautiful people are beautiful from their skin to their hair to their muscle tone to their sleep patterns. Unhealthy people often give the appearance of imbalance, which is reflected in their skin, hair, muscles and sleep patterns. Coming back to real whole food will result in almost immediate improvement of a healthy appearance. Being a Health Beautiful person means feeding your body goodness.

No Starving Yourself, Please

Always anticipate your need for food, and never wait to feel hungry before you eat. The reason for this is that your hunger will prompt the release of hormones that tell the thyroid, brain, and various digestive organs that you are in starvation mode. The body will hang onto its backup reserves of energy and leave you feeling sluggish. Food will not be burned in the body's effort to reserve energy. Instead, energy will be stored as fat in safe places like your hips and belly.

By starving yourself, the body will start to normalize a low calorie intake by anticipating a need for the body's release of energy. As the body refuses to release energy and tries to regulate the intake of non-nutritive empty calories, it will begin to gather fat. The next time that a flurry of calories arrives, the body will store and store and store fat in every place it can. When the normalization of metabolic function occurs after being forced to repeatedly regulate the intake of empty calories, your metabolism slows down. This is how someone who eats a 1200-calorie diet may become overweight and disproportioned.

The onset of an unhealthy metabolism in response to a non-nutritive diet often results in organ fatigue, such as adrenal fatigue or pancreatic exhaustion, which may result in a medical diagnosis that requires drugs to reactivate organ function and healthy metabolic function. Unfortunately, the effect of these drugs on the body can be harsh and damaging over long periods of time. The persistence of inflammation is the cause of most diseases, but poor diet causes the majority of inflammation in the first place.

When working with a client who wants to lose weight, I always examine what they are eating; however, my focus is mainly on what they are not eating. More often than not, the client who holds onto weight and restricts calories is not eating enough nutrient-rich food. In many cases they rely on starvation for weight control. By educating them on the benefits of real food and introducing meals that provide more energy, my clients reverse the slowdown of their metabolism and begin to feel more comfortable around food. They begin to associate good feelings with good quality food. The change in their mindset from restriction to nourishment changes everything for them.

Trust that your food selection is the most important aspect of weight loss, not starvation. Being a Health Beautiful person means being conscious of your own responsibility to yourself in nourishing your body with good food. Nourishment *will* make you Health Beautiful.

Set a Goal, Meet a Goal

Defining what you want is important for reaching your goals. Knowing why you want it will help to get you there.

Food that contains information that the body needs will make you the perfect size for your genetic makeup. Keep in mind that you don't need to be a certain number on the scale or size in jeans. Goals that focus on weight and size are difficult for lots of reasons. Striving for good nutrition instead is easy and immediate– you can accomplish your goals with every meal.

Fill your plate with real and highly nutritious food and you will lose weight. Your meal design is completely within your control. Setting goals that encourage small, easily met and rewarding outcomes is the most effective way to make changes for the better. Seeking goals that are hard to reach and difficult to measure will leave you feeling stressed and unhappy. Almost every one of my clients expresses striving for happiness as a real goal; they want to be happy with themselves and happy with their life every day.

Serving your body what it needs based on your life's demands.

For example, it is breakfast time and you need an abundance of energy for a long series of tennis matches with your tennis club.

What do you serve yourself?

- ✓ Serve yourself energy with long-burning complex carbohydrates
- ✓ Antioxidants for cell perfection, ready to activate and receive nutrition
- ✓ Omega fatty acids for cognitive function and concentration
- ✓ Protein to repair muscles
- ✓ Natural sugar sources for stimulation

The perfect breakfast to prepare for this activity is homemade oatmeal with fresh berries, sunflower seeds and a drizzle of maple syrup. The nutritional content of this meal is perfect for an active day ahead.

The meal described above is an example of how I educated one of my clients to address her physical needs, based on her activities. I taught her what nutritional benefits certain foods would offer her to perform at her very best. Eventually, she was able to develop her own meals based on her activities each day going forward. A smaller goal of hers was to enjoy her tennis game and be proud of her performance on the court. She achieved this goal through meeting nutritional demands before her body required them. Weight loss was a side effect to this person's goal to be a better tennis player. Supporting her nutritional needs in order to support her tennis goals resulted in weight loss.

Vegetables at Every Meal

Fill your plate with vegetables every chance you get. To maximize the nutritious benefits of vegetables, focus on variety. A large variety of vegetables improves gut microbiome diversity, and as a result your metabolic health may improve. They should be as natural as possible. This means the kind of vegetables that grow in a garden or on an organic farm, not the prepackaged kind or a powder of pulverized produce meant to be added to a smoothie.

The makeup of a vegetable is such that, when it reacts with your digestive system starting in the mouth, strong bonds (the precursors to antigens, which promote T-cell activity) are created. These are absorbed by the body and used to do many things, such as protecting you from illness, producing energy, healing on the microscopic level, aiding respiration, letting the heart beat and blood flow with ease, keeping a balanced rhythm of hormone release and sleep, producing antibodies and facilitating a regulated metabolism.

This impressive list of health benefits explains why I want my vegetables. I want my heart to beat with ease and my sleep to come naturally. I want my body to fight off disease and repel unnecessary fat. I want to have a thyroid that functions as it should, prompting the right levels of hormones to be released at the right times. I will stop at nothing to guarantee that I have done everything in my power to set myself up for health, so that I can live my life with power.

Vegetables work best as the main event of a meal, not on the side as an afterthought. For a truly healthy meal, 75% of the plate should be covered with a variety of perfectly cooked or raw vegetables. A wide variety of vegetables offers a wide variety of nutrients. Some vegetables carry a huge abundance of highly beneficial vitamins, minerals and proteins. Kale is one example. But don't stop at kale for your vitamins and minerals. Variety in the daily diet is an important way to be in the best health possible.

Different food reacts differently within your body, yielding varying results. For example, potassium-rich foods support cell equilibrium. The maintenance of fluids helps to prevent everything from leg cramps and muscle fatigue to blood pressure and kidney disease. Good sources of potassium are found in a wide variety of vegetables, including beans, squash and cauliflower. The FDA recommends that you get about 3500 milligrams of potassium per day, but you probably won't want to eat beans at every single meal just because they contain potassium.[9]

Use your senses to find the freshest foods and select a variety to fulfill your needs for vitamins and minerals. We crave variety in our food for a reason! By serving dark, leafy, cooked vegetables such as kale alongside light, crisp vegetables such as endive, you cover all of your bases. By eating an abundance of varied vegetables, you ensure that your nutritional needs are always met and disease is kept at bay.

Your health relies on nutrients found most abundantly in vegetables. A low-carb, meat-heavy diet, supplemented with powdered protein and 100-calorie bags of junk food, will not make you healthy. This lifestyle typically leads to profound illness and disease. What will help you to realize the goal of achieving a healthy body is eating real food that was grown in the earth, throughout the day, every day. The body needs the nutritional information and will work perfectly when served what it needs. It's simple— give your body what it needs and it won't have to work extra hard to give you what you want.

Breaking Bad... Habits

Your body is made up of cells that read information. The information comes to the cell through a complex system of coding, decoding, enzymatic reactions, and chemical relays. What you need to know is that cells depend on specific information to keep you alive and productive. When the cells do not receive the information that they need, illness will appear over time. This illness can show itself in many ways, from autoimmune disorders and diabetes to heart and thyroid disease.

Prior to the onset of serious disease, more benign symptoms appear in various ways, including acne and rashes, food sensitivities, headaches, and fatigue. The body is smart. It will try to substitute what it needs from what is supplied and will exploit that resource for as long as it is available. When your body does not receive the required information in the form of good nutrition, it is tapped out. That is when the real danger strikes. The body (which has been deprived of nutrition for too many years and in its place was fed chemically-processed food that cells cannot use or tap into for information) becomes diseased. The bad news is, once disease has settled in, it becomes very difficult to dislodge.

Through poor eating habits, the body has been deprived of the information needed to function properly. The body will lose its ability to compensate for poor nutritional information, as in pancreatic exhaustion, which results in pre-diabetic symptoms and eventually leads to type 2 diabetes. The medicine that has been prescribed to make up for the body's inability to function properly is very effective for alleviating these symptoms, yet these medications are very costly and can have various detrimental side effects. Medicating preventable diseases is not a solution for your health. More often than not, the medicated person's desire is to be free from prescription drugs and able to maintain their health on their own.

Breaking bad eating habits and reversing the onset of disease can be very challenging. This is where I help my clients the most. In my practice, the client is encouraged to rethink everything that he or she eats and to recognize that his or her body reacts to food in ways that are unique to the individual. A one-size-fits-all food plan doesn't work.

My clients are always surprised by how simple it is to be healthy. The closer you look at the relationship between food and illness, the simpler it becomes. I educate people about what their bodies need and how to fulfill those needs. Feeling great and being thin and strong are the side effects of regaining their health. Seeing my clients establish health and lose their illness is one of the most wonderful rewards in my profession.

90/10 Living

Please take a moment to think about the last meal that satisfied you, the kind of meal that sent a sensation of fulfillment and fuel throughout your body, that is free from emotional distress, where you know that you worshiped your body in a way that will deliver great results. "Feeling great" is how you will describe yourself when you are healthy. Think about how wonderful it will be to enjoy food and to know that you are making yourself a comfortable place in your world, filled with good feelings and great energy.

When you eat well all of the time, you feel great all of the time. Once you get over the reset process of reintroducing goodness into your body and ridding the body of chemicals and dependence on processed convenience food, once you have gotten over your addictions to food that does not serve your needs, and once you have created an inner balance where you can rely on specific results based on specific meals you have served your Health Beautiful body, this is the most amazing feeling.

I eat to serve my needs and I can rely on my food to deliver exactly what I am looking for at any given moment. Consider this: When you drink a cup of coffee you feel a certain way, and when you take a drink of wine you feel a different way. Food that does not contain stimulants or depressants like caffeine and alcohol the same thing, just more subtly. If you want energy from your food, you need to eat food with energy-producing qualities. If you are eating food that depletes your energy, then you will feel tired and in some situations you might even experience a "food coma," or extreme tiredness that leaves you unable to function for hours. Being Health Beautiful is being able to rely on your own judgment to deliver everything that your body and your life require of you.

Living a 90/10 life will deliver the results that make you Health Beautiful. Every item of food that comes across your plate offers an opportunity to be healthy. This is not a far-off state of existence. Being healthy is something that happens as the result of all of your choices. When you decide not to smoke, you are choosing to live healthily. If you add a full plate of vegetables rather than a small side of vegetables to your meal, you have decided to eat healthily. If you drink water and move your body, you have made a decision to be healthy. The act of eating an orange rather than a cookie is being healthy.

Getting on the scale does not make you healthy. Talking about how you are going to make changes doesn't make you healthy. We encounter opportunities to take various paths throughout our lives. Adults understand that certain paths may result in specific rewards, and other paths may lead to more punishing outcomes. A night of binge-drinking results in a hangover and possible social dilemmas that unraveled during the binge. Eating a plate of vegetables results in energy and fortification of your health that is far-reaching.

As you make more and more healthy choices, the results will become clearer and more apparent. The healthier you are, the healthier you feel because your body develops a balance and a reliable recognition of food as information. The balance that I speak of is one where you put information into your body on a regular basis, and your body anticipates that it will be served what it requires to meet its needs for high quality nutrition. A dependable source of nutrients results in higher performance output by the body. You know that saying, "you only get out of something what you put into it?" It's true.

The human body is designed to protect itself at all costs.

When your body can rely on good information all the time, it will release excess fat and inflammation. Fat and inflammation are the results of confusion within the body. Fat and inflammation are created when the body is stressed. A stressed body is the result of poor nutrition. The symptoms may vary but the cause is the same. As you begin to feed yourself healthy food all the time, your organs function with ease and you can rely on improved energy and a general feeling of vitality.

It takes a consistent source of healthy food to run your body well. This is why I recommend a 90/10 lifestyle. A lot of health plans fail because they do not emphasize the reality that healthy living is an ongoing process. You cannot eat like a bird, pecking on tasteless raw vegetables all day, and then binge on pretzels and large plates of cheese-smothered fried food at night, and expect positive results. That behavior does not create a reliable balance that your body can depend on. You will achieve the best results when you take every meal and every snack as an opportunity to give yourself the best nutrition possible. You will create a balance, a consistency of nourishment that results in inner strength and outward health.

As you increase the nutritional content of your meals, you will start to look at food differently. You will start to examine what your food offers your body. You will not want to contaminate the delivery of nourishment with confusing chemicals or genetically altered food. You will want to deliver a perfect meal, filled to the brim with great information. This will serve to improve your outward appearance. Your outward appearance improves with excellent reliable energy and perfect sleep. Your skin glows, you have a flat stomach, and your muscles look toned and lean. Your "body in balance" eventually becomes the perfect shape and size that it is meant to be. You're able to bound out of bed and live your day without pain and discomfort. Automatically, when you can rely on your healthy physical being, your emotional being improves. Your confidence soars because you know in your heart that your body is perfect. Your body has become perfectly Health Beautiful. This is 90% of the 90/10 lifestyle.

Now for the other 10%:

I challenge myself daily, trying to make each plate of food serve a specific nutritional need. I try to see if I can have a fully nutritious plate of food– a plate that not only serves me but contains nothing but food that serves my needs. I try to never consume food that does not serve my needs. Having said that, I am a person who lives in a world filled with temptation and where some foods won't serve all of my needs.

Take a plate of pasta, for example. There is not a single element of benefit in that plate, other than taste. I like pasta, and I like including it in my weekly menu, so I'll allow it and less nutritive foods like it to comprise no more than 10% of my diet. I'll use pasta as a vehicle for delivering other foods, like vegetables. I will have rigatoni with homemade tomato sauce, sautéed kale and mushrooms. I smother my pasta with vegetables. They take up at least 75% of my plate. The pasta is the side and the vegetables are the main dish. I love these meals because they satisfy a craving for carbohydrates and fulfill my nutritional needs with nutrient-dense vegetables.

Confidence in my choice of mostly vegetables with a side of pasta allows for a positive outpouring of emotion towards my food. 10% is the maximum allotment of food that does not meet your nutritional needs, according to this plan. When you add something void of nutritional value or even detrimental to the functionality of other nutrients that you've already ingested, it should not be significantly detrimental to your health. This is because you have systems within your body that regulate, filter and purify your blood, which counteract the influx of chemicals and carcinogenic substances that we are exposed to on a regular basis.

These systems work perfectly when they are relied upon in

small doses and activated to purify the body only a small amount of the time. When someone constantly eats a diet filled with chemicals, the body becomes exhausted and you may experience bizarre symptoms of irregularity like adrenal fatigue or thyroid disease. I encourage you to learn from this book that your body will give you perfection if you feed it perfect food. Your systems work optimally only when given the opportunity to do so. Keeping away from processed food will result in a clean and highly productive metabolic output.

Imagine and Realize Your Own Wellbeing

Love yourself enough to take care of your own wellbeing by making the executive decision to take control of your life through nutrition. This will propel you and your family towards happiness.

Imagine a life where you are no longer restrained by the chains of medication for basic functions. Envision setting out into the world with confidence that your body will react as you need it to all day long.

Believe that you can live without the fear of food and how your body reacts to it. You don't have to question the calorie content because you have simplified your food and you know what makes you feel good. Likewise, you know which foods to avoid because certain ingredients cause adverse reactions that you are aware of.

What does being healthy mean to you? Is it daunting or even incomprehensible to imagine life without the restraint of being sick? Can you dream about sleeping through the night and breathing easily without medication? Is it scary to imagine a day without medicine or a night without sedatives? Can you picture your life without allergies? Is it possible to make it through winter after winter without a cold?

Yes, it *is* possible to be this healthy– people do it all the time. I often go years without any colds or illness. I may get a stuffy nose or spend a day or two feeling a little tired and under the weather, but I get back to normal quickly and without medication. The difference between this response and being sick for the longer term is an optimally functioning and highly effective immune system that is continuously strengthened by good nutritional choices.

Being sick with a cold is not the end of the world, but it's an amazing feeling to be able to avoid poor health as often as possible. Have faith that your body can heal itself, by itself. Dr. Andrew Weil emphasizes the importance of a "springy immunity."[10] In his books and lectures, he repeatedly talks about how one's immune response of fever and temporary inflammation is perfectly normal and welcome in the body's effort to fight off illness. Fever becomes a problem only when it is sustained over a long period of time.

Fever is a normal reaction to infection. I'm not talking about a high delirious fever or fever-induced seizures– these require medical attention. I am talking about the low-grade fever that you get that makes you feel achy all over and sends you to bed. This is good news. This means the body is doing what it needs to do to fight off the virus it has contracted. Research shows that raised body temperature increases the activity of a virus fighting T-cell called CD-8. When body temperature rises, the T-cell is activated and fights off the virus. The study also showed that the activation of lymphocyte-like T-cells improves the functionality of your body's immune system.[11] Understanding that your body has perfect responses already in place to protect you is an essential part of being healthy. By taking fever-lowering medications, you interrupt your own body's immune system. You suppress what the body needs to fight off the cold and to build immunity for your next encounter with a cold or infection.

Your body will heal itself by itself if you give it a chance. Our bodies have complex built-in immune responses to infections, invasive bacteria, viruses, and disease. The use of antibiotics has been shown to destroy the body's natural defense bacteria in the gut. In cases where antibiotics were given, much of the delicate beneficial microbiota in our gut, which maintains and supports our immune health, is killed and may not fully recover after treatment.[12] This is potentially dangerous because we rely on our immune systems to protect us from diseases and viruses. When our immunity is compromised by antibiotic use, we lower our resistance to illness.

Taking the time and trusting the body to respond and heal itself is important for maintaining great health for years into the future. In addition to susceptibility to dangerous viruses and invasive bacteria, antibiotic use is directly linked to intestinal inflammation-related diseases. It all boils down to supporting the gut microbiome with dietary fiber and avoiding compromising the balance within your gut unless you are in a life-threatening situation. Keeping calm and being aware of your health and your illnesses are all vital elements of your Health Beautiful life.

As a parent, I had to learn this lesson myself. When my kids were very young, ages four and six, my younger son Jamie contracted a virus that lead to a high fever. He lay in bed and I gave him over-the-counter fever-reducing medicine. He leapt into a delusional, delirious state where he was hallucinating and speaking in a bizarre voice. We called the doctor and hovered over him, hoping that the fever would go down and that he would return to normal. This behavior was repeated two times. We took him to a neurologist who studied his brain and neurological stats, to determine whether he had been having seizures. He was absolutely fine. All of his blood work and tests came back normal.

About two months later, Jamie had a cough so I gave him an over-the-counter cough suppressant. It happened again. What we thought was a fever-induced reaction that had caused his bizarre behavior before turned out to be a reaction to the children's fever and cough suppressants. This was upsetting and disturbing because we trust in pharmaceutical companies to provide us with medication that takes care of us. We trust in the medical community to keep us well. Both failed my little boy repeatedly.

In addition to suppressing fevers and coughs, the medication also caused side effects that I never thought were possible. As Jamie was going through this ordeal, we all were so afraid for him. He was like a delicate egg that I felt that I had to handle carefully as we tried to uncover what was happening to him. I believe I instinctively knew that there was an environmental cause for his behavior. I was reminded of my own experiences with food and artificial ingredients that made me fall ill as a young child, and thought of how the same thing could be happening to Jamie. When we received the results telling us that all tests were normal and that he was not suffering from a brain disorder or other disease, I was relieved of course, but I still lacked an explanation for his behavior. It is very difficult to disregard medical advice like that regarding the supposed safety of fever-reducing medicine that is advertised on television.

Advertised medicine is branded in such a way that we believe that we are harming our kids if we do *not* administer it to them. It was finally a relief when, with the diligent persistence of our pediatrician who resists prescribing medication unless absolutely necessary, we determined that the over-the-counter medications were triggering Jamie's odd reactions. I thought it was so sad that it took such extreme circumstances to uncover what I personally had experienced as a young child in my own child. Trusting an instinct to hesitate to give unnecessary chemicals to your kids is imperative. I believe educating yourself about the pros and cons of medical intervention for common ailments is a mandatory part of parenting.

Now, when my son shows symptoms of a cold, I stop and think about what is going on with him. I don't let fear take hold of me when he gets a little sick. I watch and listen to what is happening. What works best is sleep, soup and love, an open window and bundling up in warm blankets. This we know to work because his colds usually only last for one or two days. Luckily, these days he doesn't get sick often. We go to well visits at the doctor for his yearly checkup and are delighted to find him healthy and developing on schedule with each yearly visit.

We are usually congratulated by our pediatrician for having a healthy year because we have often not seen our doctor since the last well visit the previous year. It is almost like a medal of honor that we all wear. We are well. We aren't sick and we get better when we do get sick. This is total control over our health.

This immune response that we have here at the Kretschmer house is being Health Beautiful in the very best way. We have great immunity. Believe me– I am so very grateful for our gene pool and our ability to respond to our health as we want to. We care for our health in ways that promote our bodies' immune response to work at its best. I do understand that not every family has the luxury to live this way. I had to deal with illness that seemed out of my control as a child and I have had to do the same as a parent and as a spouse. It is frightening, a difficulty that I wish could be eradicated for everyone. Some of our friends and family are burdened with immune-compromised illnesses and we see how tough it is on them to sustain their health.

What I would like you to take away from this is that we often rush to suppress a mild temperature or cough with over-the-counter medication without questioning why. You do not have to just accept that you are sick. Some illness is brought on through neglect of your own health. Some illness is due to your body's total rejection of certain foods or medications, or the result of damage caused by medication and prolonged neglect.

There are many professional healers who are very informed and well versed in the intricate relationships between your gut and your symptoms. I stress that, if this is your issue, be aware that the symptom alerts you to the problem. Solve the problem and the symptom will disappear. Mask the symptom and the problem may transform into a larger, compounded medical condition. By taking charge of your health, you face the fact that your own actions may be the very thing that caused your health problems in the first place. Educating yourself and being proactive about solving those problems is an essential and necessary part of being Health Beautiful.

Health is Measured by Little Buggers

Your health depends on the living organisms that are inside your body and on the surface of your skin. Without these bacteria you cannot survive. There are approximately ten times more bacterial cells in and on the body than human cells.[13] The microbiome differs greatly from one individual to the next, and these microbes work to keep you alive. Usually, the healthier a person is, the more diverse and populous the microorganisms contained within their gut tend to be.[14]

Researchers are currently attempting to discover ways to improve and protect an individual's gut microbiome.[15] Keeping the gut microbiome healthy is done through everything from vaginal birth and breastfeeding, to keeping in contact with the environment around you (including pets and soil from your garden), and using soap instead of antibacterial cleansers on your hands.[16] Reserving antibiotic use for treating serious bacterial infections that can only be cured with such measures is recommended by the researchers in this field because the gut microbiome is in danger when antibiotics are administered.[17]

Antibiotics wipe out large parts of the microbiome and you are left susceptible to viruses and colds, as well as other types of infection. Replenishing the healthy bacteria through targeted nutrition with a variety of microbes found in various probiotics needs to be a priority in this case. Different probiotics replenish different cultures of bacteria. I recommend consulting with the well-informed staff of a health food store (or a pharmacist) who can guide you to specific products. Simultaneously, heal the damage done to the gut by antibiotics through the use of a daily dose of fermented foods, such as kimchi or sauerkraut (not the cooked variety– labels usually state "contains live cultures").

We can help to keep our gut microbiomes healthy by eating dietary fiber, which provides the polysaccharides these little guys thrive on.[18] Dietary fiber is found mainly in vegetables and real whole grains, not whole grain bread produced from milled flour with the fiber and nutrients put back in, but whole grains prepared and consumed in their natural state.

One of my favorite exercises that I conduct with my clients is exposing them to the loveliness of whole grains. This is where so many people fall short. Many people that seek out my services are in terrific health, but they are looking to expand on their culinary skills to further their health in natural ways. I recommend a trip to a healthy supermarket that has a section where various grains, seeds, nuts, and dried fruit are sold loosely in bulk.

I suggest that they experiment with serving a new grain each day until they discover which ones they enjoy and which they may prefer to pass on. Many love to add grains such as amaranth and quinoa to their meals, as these are very easy and quick to prepare. My Italian heritage draws me toward faro, an ancient grain used in parts of Africa and Italy for centuries. I use and recommend buckwheat (a gluten-free grain, unrelated to wheat) and kamut berries, which come from wheat and thus contain gluten.

Whole grains are extremely high in fiber and are an excellent source of protein. Grains are complex carbohydrates in their most health-promoting form. The anatomy of a whole grain supplies certain forms of fiber that, when digested, are beneficial to cardiovascular health and provide a source of long-lasting energy. When consumed whole, grains offer a nutty, earthy taste and add terrific texture to meals. Exploring and including grains and seeds in your meals to replace white rice and sandwich bread is strongly encouraged and should be part of any heart healthy, gut healthy, and energy healthy diet.

Eating peas and carrots alone will not provide the necessary diversity of nutrients and fiber required for good health. A highly diverse vegetable- and whole grain-based diet helps to support a highly diverse gut microbiome. It has been shown that healthy, strong people tend to have more diverse microbes in their guts, suggesting a clear connection between a healthy gut microbiome and healthy eating habits.[19,20]

This is so very interesting to me because I am supremely satisfied with vegetable-centric meals. Afterwards, I don't feel sick or experience digestive unrest. I sleep better and have loads of energy. I don't get sick often and when I do, I get better quickly. When eating a vegetable-heavy diet, what's most surprising to me is that I feel totally satisfied as I eat. I experience the flipping of a switch that turns off the desire to continue eating (which is not something that I experience when eating lasagna).

To me, eating a large plate of vegetables for lunch is far more satisfying than a turkey and cheese sandwich. At some point my brain will say "stop eating" and I will not feel hunger or the need to consume any other food for several hours. This is because I have given my body all the necessary information it needs at that time. The challenge for many people is breaking the habit of grabbing a cold cut sandwich in favor of selecting a vegetable plate for lunch. Fostering health on a microscopic level within your body has far-reaching benefits.

So what should you do with this information? You now know that every part of your biological existence is affected by your unique microbial makeup, and healthy individuals have more diversity and higher populations of microbes in their bodies. You also learned that bacteria live on dietary fiber found in whole grains and vegetables in their natural, unprocessed state. The purpose of this book is to teach you how your body reacts to and depends on healthy food. It is up to you to improve what is currently deficient in your life so that you can live in a Health Beautiful world.

   Many of the articles cited in this discussion are part of *The Human Microbiome Project Collection*, an ongoing scientific effort to explore and understand human microbial diversity.[21] If you suffer from persistent unresolved symptoms or repetitive illness, I encourage you to explore the cited studies to further understand what may be contributing to your particular imbalance.

Boost Nutrition and Enjoy the Results

Planning ahead and eating before you are feeling hungry, and eating vegetables with every meal, will help you to get healthy, be skinny and stay the perfect weight for your body type. The perfect you is happy with your choices, and calm about your relationship with food and how it affects you. The perfect you feels pleasure rather than guilt about food choices, and has confidence in these selections. The perfect you is clear about what great nourishment provides to your body.

Even when making occasional choices to be indulgent, you still convey a good feeling to yourself that you were in control of your decisions. You planned and prepared to serve yourself with indulgences, recognizing that you have cravings. The very healthy individual eats extremely good quality and highly nutritious food. The very healthy individual's body balances its function, normalizing and responding easily to the demands life poses on the body. Being in great health allows you to live and work easily by supporting your body with nutrition and love.

It's not about giving up sugar, carbs or gluten, although these restrictions may make you feel better. It is the addition of highly nutritious food that yields results. If you look at food as information for the cells, you will choose food that is nourishing. That nourishment will allow the body to function at its peak. Therefore, if you do reintroduce sugar, gluten, salt and other elements, your organ systems will all be working as they should and will be able to siphon out the bad chemicals and substances, like excess sugar in one meal or extra salt in another. Meanwhile, the well-nourished body is able to digest and absorb information from the food that you've eaten. The liver will clean your blood and your heart will pump with ease. Rashes will not appear because there are no chemical overloads for your body to deal with, and the pounds will disappear.

Imagine...

- Being your perfect body size and shape *as nature and genetics intended for you*
- Having the energy to make a difference in your life
- Being free from medical dependence
- Being happy with your life
- Being confident in your own skin

How Food Makes You Feel

How does the food that you eat make you feel?

Please take a moment to think back on the last five nights. After you ate dinner, how did you feel? Make a list of every emotion and every physical response that you had towards dinner.

Questions to prompt this exercise:

- How did you anticipate or plan each dinner?
- When did you eat?
- What type of setting were you in during the meal?
- Who was with you?
- How was your mood while you prepared and ate your food?
- What did you feel physically after dinner?
- Were you satisfied or just stuffed?
- Were you energized or in a food coma?
- How was the rest of your evening?
- Did you celebrate your meal and choices?
- Were you guilt-ridden about your gluttony?
- Did you experience regret?
- Did you experience pride?
- Did you go for extra snacks later?
- How many additional drinks did you have later?
- Did you sleep soundly or restlessly?
- How was your digestion the next day?
- Did your food serve your nutritional and energy needs?

There was a time in my life when I would feel sick, tired, and desperately in need of a bed every night after dinner. I would feel guilty, and angry about my lack of discipline when eating. My head would swim with declarations of willpower to do better tomorrow. I would lay plans to stop eating seconds and skip the wine and have self-control when choosing carbs. I would beat myself up and look for excuses for my behavior. The next day, boom! I experienced the same scenario. It was a terrible time in my life.

I hated the way food made me feel. I had negative feelings towards food, both emotionally and physically. I hated the belly that I had and the bra strap rolls that I felt I needed to cover. I never, ever ate a meal and said, "Wow, I feel great!" afterwards. I never made a dinner that gave me energy. All of my food tasted terrific, though. I am an excellent cook and I love to make food and share it with others.

The problem was simple: I was not nourishing my body with vitamins and minerals. I was barely eating good fats, found in seeds and avocados. I still believed that I might get fat from eating fat. I held onto the false notion that less food meant less weight, and made my struggle about willpower over food rather than becoming a healthy person. I was counting calories. I was focused on how I looked, not how I felt. I ate along with the crowd and consumed food that did not serve my needs. I had a negative relationship with food. Sadly, my self-esteem was bound by the chains of destructive emotions that fueled my lack of willpower. Thank goodness that is over.

Choosing food that makes you feel great

When I am working with clients in our first session, we establish goals for their health. Often, the main goal is to lose weight.

Client: "My goal is to lose ten pounds."

I interrupt and set guidelines for their goals. Losing ten pounds is not a goal, it is a measurement that is not obtainable on a day-to-day basis. The struggle attached to losing weight is quite negative and defeating. Often, when I give permission to the client to stop weighing him or herself and to refocus his or her goals for feeling great, they are relived and immediately feel happier with themselves. They no longer have to battle with themselves about how they ate or didn't eat and how much they weigh. Weight goals are subjective and are hard to obtain.

I advise my clients to set health goals that can be assessed on a daily basis, goals assessed with qualitative measurements for how a meal makes them feel, not how much they weigh. There is no diet in the world that will cause you to lose weight in a day, certainly not ten pounds.

Setting the goal

- "I want to feel great."
- "I want to feel happy with my body."
- "I will be more energetic when I feel great."
- "My attitude toward food will be positive."
- "I will eat food that serves my energy, emotional, and mental needs."

By redirecting your goals towards serving your needs, you are able to reach a goal at every meal. The hook sets and you will strive to achieve that feeling of happiness, satisfaction and energy with every meal. Being able to meet goals at each meal facilitates the creation of new healthy habits that serve your needs.

The opposite is true for setting a goal to lose weight. When you set that goal, each meal feels like you have taken a step backward. This is because people associate calorie intake with gaining weight. The fact is that the number of calories is not what makes someone gain weight; it is the lack of nutritional quality found in those calories that makes a difference.

Take a moment to stop and think about what your health goals are. Do you want to lose weight? If so, please ask yourself how losing weight will make you healthy. Clarify your goals and word them in a way that expresses how you see yourself existing once you have regained your health.

- How do you feel every moment and at every meal?
- Do you work more effectively?
- Are your relationships stronger?
- How does the world look to you once you have gained energy, are no longer living with pain and can enjoy a night of restful sleep?

Resetting the mind to think about how food will serve your needs.

I teach a cooking class about snacking and deconstructing cravings. The main focus is on understanding what you need in order to satisfy cravings. Eating a particular food may not satisfy the craving. Examining the need and what you may be lacking will deliver satisfaction to your physical and emotional needs. The snack is often a filler, a poor substitute for your needs. I am not suggesting that you substitute a snack with another snack. I am suggesting that you fulfill those needs early so that you won't crave snacks that don't serve you later.

Let's say you are craving a candy bar in the afternoon. Examining what the candy will give you will uncover what you are lacking. Providing your body with what it really needs will satisfy the craving and reset your body to a balanced state. The candy bar is simple sugar and very sweet.

Something sweet

Sweet emotional cravings sometimes occur where love and kindness are lacking.

Calling and sharing loving words with your sweetie is a great idea when you experience these cravings. Find a way to laugh out loud, perhaps a funny video on the internet. A hug or even love in the afternoon will satisfy your sweet emotional cravings.

Sweet energy cravings are also related to lack of sleep.

Almost every single client that I have ever worked with was suffering from a lack of restful rejuvenating sleep when we first started. Sweet foods provide quick energy and the brain knows it. Craving a candy bar at 2 p.m. when you have been awake since 6 a.m. is perfectly natural.

Scheduling a ten minute power nap at this time of low energy is ideal. The *Huffington Post* established napping rooms and increased their productivity within the office as a result. Although not every company is progressive enough to have napping rooms, getting proper sleep will help to deter sweet cravings later in the day. Long, restful sleep at night restores your metabolic needs. These are the most vital needs in the body, the ones that deal with cell reconstruction and organ rest and repair. When these are satisfied properly, the cravings for energy (a.k.a. sweets) will subside.

Sweet cravings indicate a lack of fuel

The body gets energy from three sources: fat, carbohydrates, and sleep. When those needs are not met, that tired, sluggish feeling occurs. By eating a lunch that includes high quality fats, you will meet your body's need for long-burning energy that is utilized later in the day. Some of my clients learned to have two small lunches that are good sources of energy to relieve their cravings for sweets. Having an omelet with avocado at 11 a.m. and a sweet potato between 2 and 3 p.m. is a perfect example of this. Eating proper fat as fuel to start the day also diminishes cravings for sweets.

Sweet cravings indicate a starving body

Craving sweets in the late afternoon is a symptom of a lack of nutrition. The dangers of eating less food than one needs can be made apparent to everyone if they would just pause and look at what they are *not* giving themselves. By eating a handful of cereal and then working out, then eating a tasteless salad made with nothing but cucumbers, you have not nourished the body with the energy and nutrients that it requires via carbohydrates, fat, vitamins, and minerals. Messages are sent to the brain that there is a need for energy. The brain associates sweetness with energy, which explains your candy bar craving.

Eating entire meals that include good fats and long-burning carbohydrates helps to curb cravings for sweets. Long-burning carbohydrates include whole grains and seeds in their natural state, not bread or white rice. Faro and brown rice are two excellent examples. The anatomy of a grain is complex. When it is manipulated into flour or otherwise processed out of its natural state, this alters how your body reacts to that energy source. The complexities of these biochemical reactions are fascinating, but I will reserve those biochemistry lessons for another setting.

Addictive sweets cravings

The sad fact is that the brain is highly susceptible to addiction to sweets and refined simple sugars, which are absorbed directly into the bloodstream and not utilized by the normal metabolic processes. Food items that contain sucrose and fructose are very addictive and cause most cravings for sweetened food or beverages.[22,23]

Making significant changes to one's diet by switching to highly digestible sugars like pure honey and maple syrup will help to decrease sugar cravings throughout the day. Choosing food with energy early in the day will help you to pass up the candy later. Another strategy you can employ is leaving your work environment and stepping outside, because taking deep breaths of fresh air will distract the brain enough for you to gain control of the cravings. Training yourself to satisfy cravings with healthy actions rather than destructive ones empowers your decision-making ability and strengthens your conviction, enabling you to meet your goals.

Honest examination of what your habits do to fuel your cravings is the most important step toward making your goals happen.

I was working with a company where the CEO wanted me to educate the staff about healthy eating habits. Within the first week, one of the managers told me that he was addicted to the candy bowl at work. He would get tired around two o'clock and walk over to the break room where there was a large bowl perpetually filled with snacks. I proposed that the break room be a sweets-free environment and management agreed. No one was permitted to bring any sugary sweets like candy, cookies, cakes, or donuts to the mutual workspace. Some staff members resisted at first, but management could not ignore the rising number of diabetics in the office. The physical health of the employees was deteriorating, partly because of the unhealthy foods so readily available within the office environment.

The break room sweets were literally making people sick and costing the company money in health care costs and missed work. After removing unhealthy snacks from the office, it only took a week for this man to reset his cravings and serve his needs.

Look at your environment, at home and at your workplace– are you providing addictive substances to yourself, your family or your coworkers that fuel unhealthy cravings?

Through an honest examination of your food and how it makes you feel, you can create goals that reflect what you really want from food. Don't be afraid to eat real food. Convenience created by pre-packaged food leads to a disconnect between you and your food. Every meal does not need to be a five course gourmet dinner; it is perfectly fine to keep the food as simple as possible. Staying honest and connected with your food lays the foundation for understanding how the food affects you. The association that you will make between what you eat and how you feel is essential to satisfying your health needs. When your health needs are met, weight loss will follow. Creating the cognitive connection between the goal to feel great and how to get there is a key part of fortifying your health. Understanding what you need versus what you want will give you the strength to make choices that support your health by supporting your needs.

Feeling great in a pair of jeans or having the energy to race around the park with your kids are the positive side effects of setting yourself up with a diet rich in highly nutritious food. When you eat highly nutritious food, you will naturally become thinner, stronger and more energetic. Meeting this goal with each meal satisfies your physical needs and your emotional cravings. Your specific cravings are very different from your neighbor's cravings. The intensive personal discussions that I conduct with each client reveal how each individual might deal with cravings in their lives.

Reducing cravings requires a great deal of honesty along

with individual examination of your own strengths and where you may be lacking mastery in your life. A craving usually indicates two things: one may be a physical void, and the other may be an emotional void. Thirst indicates that your body is currently lacking water, so drinking water usually relieves this craving. Dissatisfaction in your career may result in excessive indulgence in another area of your life, such as drinking too much alcohol or nighttime eating. The overindulgence may be filling a void that appears in another aspect of your life. Each of my clients is profoundly different in how they deal with voids in their lives, and it is up to me to listen carefully and help guide them in healthy ways toward filling those negative spaces. Having balance in your nourishment allows you to cope with external challenges. Together, the balance is struck and you are Health Beautiful.

A Health Beautiful Family

When I was expecting my first son, I was hyper-particular about every single aspect of my preparation for baby. We spent hours selecting the perfect stroller (we had a grand total of six at one point!) We washed his clothes in the perfect baby detergent. We washed the floor several times a day. We made visitors confirm their health and wash their hands. I hung lovely baby photos around the house and created the safest and most loving home possible for his arrival.

I took such care because I wanted my baby to be perfect. I wanted him to be healthy and to feel loved and comfortable. I nursed him past one year. I bought the best diapers and wipes even though their purpose is more about function than prestige. I carried him around the house endlessly, catering to his every whim and need. This has not changed too much now that he is thirteen. Oh sure, I nag and yell at him a lot more, mostly about stuff like, "brush your teeth" and "make your bed, bring down your laundry and get out to the bus stop."

I love my kids so much. I want the very, very, very best for them at every moment, always. I celebrate their wonderful brilliance and athletic and musical abilities. I laugh with them and give my every breath for their happiness. I suspect that they know I would do anything for them, except sacrifice their wellbeing for convenience or an impulsive craving. I know that my teenagers are going to eat some junk food while they are away from me, but they will never get it from my hand, and it will never be paid for from my wallet.

As we sit down for a meal the entire family engages in conversation, which often includes a discussion about how this particular meal tastes, feels, looks and affects our health. My family holds nutrition up as a necessity and a privilege. We all understand that we are fortunate to have the opportunity to be selective with our food and to demand the best for each meal. We understand how exceptional our food is and that nutritious meals help to create our happy lives. We are deeply engaged with cooking and selecting food.

My kids prefer certain supermarkets over others and when they look at menus in restaurants, they order asparagus soup rather than fried mozzarella as an appetizer. My kids look forward to bringing leftovers to school, like homemade pizza with kale and beets from Meatless Monday's dinner (this is a common practice for Nick, 13). My husband, who refuses to share his food at work, receives compliments about how great his food smells when he unpacks and heats his lunch. His coworkers often end up at the deli– a far cry from homemade veggie chili.

I began cooking at the age of eleven with my grandmother, something I treasure and deeply miss now that she is gone. I learned how to enrich meals as I learned about the specific nutrients in various ingredients. I teach my family as we cook about what certain foods contain and how they support our health. I explain how protein rebuilds and repairs muscle, whole grains supply fiber and long-burning energy, and flax seeds support cognitive delivery with their omega fatty acids. Our practices at home are an ongoing education for the family.

As my children grow and head out into the world, this education is the foundation for great health and happy lives. We uphold our health and our food choices in my family the way some people regard their religious beliefs. It is quite similar, actually. We have established a code of conduct and an understanding of food and what it means to our family that was created with honor and high expectations. Our practices for a healthy lifestyle reward my family with vibrancy and excellent health. We know that our bodies will deliver what we expect from them, as long as we have respect for the needs of our bodies. This is my Health Beautiful family, and I love them.

A Health Beautiful family has vitality and a beautiful glow that emanates from within. The children are able to concentrate and retain information in school. The adults are strong and confident. A balance has been created between work and home life. The children get quality sleep, and the adults have a healthy relationship with the kids. The Health Beautiful family recognizes their physical and mental needs and strives to provide these needs with nourishment. This family looks to enrich their lives with success. The family eats healthy food and the kids look for quality in their food selection. This family eats together and plays together. They support one another and communicate in positive ways. Activities are always on the calendar, even days of relaxation where we stay in and lounging around together. There is balance and respect for their own bodies and the wellbeing of the entire family.

The Health Beautiful family is any collection of people that fulfills this description. No matter the shape or the size that your family takes, food is the common thread running through each person. Food can be a catalyst for commonality within families that are in a state of unrest and crisis, too. Since food is a necessity and the very comfortable feeling of being well fed is part of our biological-emotional connection, it can be the thing that all members can respect and expect from each other. Making the decision to make quality food a staple in your home is an act of love.

Form Lasting Bonds While Washing the Veggies

In my practice, I sometimes lecture large groups of culturally-diverse people who work for large corporations. I once spoke in Brooklyn in front of a group of mostly women who work for a nonprofit child welfare agency. I was lecturing about how to instill the value of quality food in your kids and family members.

In the front row was a woman who was nodding her head in agreement as I spoke. She acknowledged the power of the practice of gathering her family to cook together. I was giving examples of how to draw in the kids and get them to eat real food. Not everyone has a large high tech kitchen, but everyone has a sink. You can gather your kids to stand hip-to-hip with you at the sink, washing the vegetables. The trust and confidence that you provide to your family members is immeasurable for their health. Connecting positive feelings to productive actions, and responsibilities to everyday tasks like cooking, is a valuable method for establishing honor around cooking.

I reminisced about how I stood this way with my own grandmother as a child, cooking in tiny kitchens together and learning her recipes, experiencing quality time together and making memories that I cherish every day. This type of practice, where the kids stand on a stool and wash the herbs while you prepare another part of the meal, is laying the foundation for a fundamental practice within their souls–prepping and cooking your own food for your family is valuable, and it constitutes a display of love. Whether you are a new parent or a seasoned one, this can be a first step towards creating your Health Beautiful family. If you live alone, I encourage you to find a friend and practice this sharing of food and love with them.

Creating an environment for the Health Beautiful family must include certain criteria, where food quality and healthy communication is an honored practice. A close-knit supportive relationship, where each person knows and helps the other with their weaknesses, is emphasized here. People who support you when you need help or find a reason to celebrate you when you are successful should be a part of your Health Beautiful family. Look to include the Health Beautiful family in all areas of your world that can support great health.

The workplace is a wonderful starting point for a healthy lifestyle. Many people spend most of their days with their coworkers and rely on each other for sustained productivity. Creating an environment for good quality energy and expectations for nutritious food will support quality work. Being around highly productive people will improve both your personal and professional life.

Sometimes I encourage people at my talks to have a frank conversation with loved ones or coworkers about how certain behaviors weaken their health. If your coworkers bring in cookies and set them out on the table and you are unable to resist them, this person needs to know that, although well intended and coming from a loving place, their offerings are dangerous for your health. If they want to share, please ask them to do so with healthy foods. It may seem like an imposition, yet it is the second most prevalent complaint that I hear from my clients.

Many of the people in my clients' lives don't initially support their choices to be healthy. It may be a spouse that brings home cake or a coworker who brings in donuts, but either way a conversation usually brings attention to the problem and most make the switch happily. I always use the example of smoking. If a coworker was smoking and you were experiencing respiratory illness as a result, they would be required to stop. The surprise that sometimes results from having these conversations may be that you find support from a friend or family member that you never thought would join you in your quest for health.

I once worked with a group of women who were trying to lose the thirty pounds that they had each gained since starting work at their company. There were several people at this company who were providing an endless supply of cake, cookies and candy to the employees as a gesture of "love." Unfortunately, people were getting sick and becoming frustrated with their well-meaning coworkers. This was causing a rift and creating unexpressed frustration between some of the employees. Together, we had a frank talk with the suppliers of the sweet treats and we asked them to stop. We asked that they respect that their coworkers needed love in the form of healthy support, not sweets. Once the practice ended, the work environment changed significantly. I started to see cut up fruit, bags of fresh spinach, and organic sunflower seeds around the office. It became a lighter and more productive space.

Your Health Beautiful family portrait may look very different than you expect at the outset. Regardless of where support occurs in your life, it is something that I encourage you to surround yourself with. As with all families, your own contribution of support is as vital as receiving it from your family.

Family Love

Realizing that the health of your family is in danger should trigger an instinctive desire to make real and lasting changes. This book is meant to help you to focus on what is necessary for excellent health. The reasons for motivation will vary between readers, but here are a few examples that might strike a chord in your gut and help you to imagine where your family can be in the future. I know this to be true for myself and my family, and I encourage you to find this hum or vibration of wellness and vitality in your own life. I know this to be true: mine is a Health Beautiful family.

The feeling of love is a powerful experience that drives the urge to keep family and friends near. This force keeps parents up at night, worried for their children's safety. With love comes worry, it's true. I am in love with three men: my husband Achim, who holds my heart and keeps my soul; my teenager Nicholas, who is the dearest, most empathetic and lovely kid (since early childhood he has always had the biggest heart); and Jamie, whose intellectual genius wraps me in laughter and amazement at his beautiful mind. I also love my dog Becky, whose never-ending loyalty and loveliness I can always count on for a good surge of joy. And I love my friends, who support me and allow me to be exactly who I need to be. I wish I could protect them all in a perfect bubble, and bring only good and wonderful things their way. We live in a world filled with danger and ugliness, and we are subjected to it every day. The health of the family and the people that I love are always on my mind.

This past year, we suffered a horrific experience. My husband had been going along, having made his healthy changes well and without incident. The week of Christmas 2014, he had to have emergency bypass surgery. He was experiencing severe chest pain for weeks. Five doctors sent him away with an incorrect diagnosis. One doctor even prescribed a medicine that may cause heart attacks, and came with a warning that states never to take it if you are experiencing chest pain.

It turned out that he had a clogged artery that was 99% closed. He was admitted to the hospital and the doctors told him he was not permitted to leave or he would most likely die. They said they rarely see this kind of arterial blockage, except post mortem. He had a triple bypass on December 26, 2014.

The year leading up to this, he was alcohol free for one year. He had been working out frequently and had lost thirty pounds. He was eating perfectly and all of his meals were highly nutritious. His EKG and blood pressure were perfect, "textbook" some doctors said. But he was pale, and his hands and feet were always cold. He was often out of breath and, in the six weeks leading up to the diagnosis and surgery, he experienced chest pain that became progressively severe.

The five doctors who examined and dismissed this seemingly healthy man clearly made some significant mistakes. They were looking at a skinny, outwardly healthy guy and ignoring his alarming symptoms of chest pain. But we knew that he was not okay. We knew this because he was very healthy otherwise. He had never experienced breathlessness or chest pain prior to this experience. He always felt terrific. Had chest pain and the inability to breathe because of poor general health been the norm for him, he would have dismissed it as being part of getting older. He would not have been alarmed and would not have persistently sought medical help. A forty-six-year-old man should be in prime condition. We caught the problem because his health was great.

He saved his life by eating well, giving up alcohol and exercising regularly. When I think about what a close call this was, it scares me. I am so incredibly grateful for his newborn heart now. The doctor who saved his life is a serious man to whom I owe everything. My husband's condition is a hereditary one, which means he is genetically predisposed to plaque buildup in his arteries. He took forty-six years to accumulate the plaque that clogged his artery, and the placement of the clogged artery made open-heart surgery a necessity. As a family, we went from seeing five totally incompetent doctors and their incorrect diagnoses to trusting a total stranger to open my husband's chest to rearrange his arteries and save his life. I had to put aside my doubts, hold onto hope and trust that he would survive.

The lesson is simple, yet profound: You have to be your own health advocate. You have to be able to read changes in your and your family's health and recognize when something is off. You need to trust your instincts when you hear an opinion that you feel is wrong. And then you need to put all of your faith into someone who can save your life or the lives of those you love. All of this is based solely on the current status of your health. If you constantly experience breathlessness, you might not identify this as a symptom of illness. If you are in pain on a regular basis, you wouldn't recognize chest pain as something new. If you are constantly having indigestion because of your diet or you live with a numb buzz all the time from alcohol and sleep aids, you would never know the difference if the reason behind these symptoms has changed. It is because of his otherwise excellent health that Achim is alive today. He is also recovering from his surgery way ahead of the curve and his prognosis is that of a new baby, perfectly healthy and raring to go.

Focus on your passion, anger, bliss, and the urge to lose your cool as you make healthy changes for your family. Begin to mentally list and analyze why you do what you do. The love that you feel for your kids, partner, parents, friends and even pets can be a wonderful source to draw energy and support from for the purpose of becoming healthier. I will even dare to add *yourself* as a motivator for getting healthy.

Finding the true love that will put meaning into this journey.

It's time to face a hard truth: The ways in which you show love for your family can be misguided, and enable the family to become sick, overweight, and tired. By keeping a steady stream of junk food in the house, parents and partners do significant damage to the health of their families. A pantry filled with junk food is disguised with good intentions. I once heard a mother of an obese child say she didn't want her kid to feel deprived, so she gives her all the food that she wants, most of which is processed junk. While she loves her kid and wants her to be happy, she has created a challenging life for her.

More than a few children suffer from this dilemma. Kids are suffering with horrible conditions and illnesses. Obesity in children is not a random disease. It is literally fed to them through poor nutrition. Pre-diabetic indicators are seen at early ages among these children, such as breasts and bellies on young boys, and acne and large bellies on young girls. Many obese kids are teased at school and they have trouble playing sports, they often have energy drops, tire in class and are more prone to getting sick. The sources are frequent takeout food, leaving for school without breakfast, and never eating a vegetable.

Having pizza several times a week and unrestrained access to processed candy and junky foods like cereal, microwave dinners, and corn syrup in everything they eat hurts these kids. The occurrence of poor health outcomes among these kids has little to do with their genetics, and everything to do with their zero nutrient diets. Parents who feed their kids this way are setting them up for shortened lives filled with lots of medication and illness. Being honest about your love toward your family and following through as an example of healthy behaviors is essential for their future.

Love is so powerful that it drives us through anything and everything, just to feel the glimmer of joy and goodness in our kids' and partners' lives. Your reason for staying the course is love. You love your kids so you cannot give them fast food today. I often will use the line, "I love you, so I won't feed you that junk."

The flipside to this is asking the same of your family, to help you meet your needs. My hope is that your family loves you as much as you love them. With this in mind, ask your family to support your nutritional needs as you gather the confidence to make great food choices. They, too, need to demand great food from the cook and the grocery shopper in the family. Asking your kids to list the family members that they love and the reasons why they love them is a wonderful way to place responsibility and power in the hands of each member. With this exercise, all of you can learn to focus on your reasons for wanting the best for each other. What is truly the best for each other may be found in good quality and nutritionally rich foods.

Engage the whole family in a real conversation about what foods are great for them. Let the kids teach you what they know. Hire a health coach to educate the family on good nutrition. A family health coach can learn about each family member's needs and coach them towards meeting those needs. I help families to redirect their focus onto what they need and where they want to go. Running behind schedule and trying to catch their breath becomes a thing of the past. Like so many families, I know what it is like to race in ten different directions, trying to hit my mark each day. I also understand that life's demands may be fulfilled with excellence when I prepare the best food possible for my family.

Knowing what your week demands from you and letting the kids acknowledge what their responsibilities are can set the stage for your meal plans. Perhaps shopping and cooking the week's meals in one day is what will work for you. I like to prep the vegetables all on the same day. I never overstuff the refrigerator. This way I know what I have and what I need. Include your kids in the meal planning and preparation. Don't allow yourself to be driven by advertisements, convenience or guilt. Require only that your meals satisfy your physical and mental demands. Thinking in terms of what you and your family need and preparing in advance may literally save their lives, and you will have a Health Beautiful family.

Spread the Love and Choose Your Food Wisely

When shopping for food, select items that serve your family's health. Please don't bring home the food that another family member struggles with. If your partner cannot say no to ice cream, don't buy it! It is really that simple. When the kids beg for waffles for breakfast, think about how their little bodies will react. Say, "No, I love you so I will give you food that will support you throughout your day." When your spouse wants to get bagels on a Sunday, tell her that you love her, and that you love yourself, and that a bagel breakfast won't serve either one of you today. Suggest that you would love a bowl of granola and fill it with beautiful berries and nuts. Remind everyone that you desire a breakfast that benefits all of you.

Yank yourself away from advertising that bombards you with sales pitches. Remember that the company selling you waffles wants you to think you are doing something good by eating their product. The ads show you pictures of kids with smiles eating waffles for breakfast. They tell you that this is a great, happy life and that you should have this waffle to make your own life this happy. They don't show you how a waffle for breakfast quickly raises your blood sugar and then makes it plummet. They don't tell you that you are setting the stage for diabetic children and fatty liver disease. They don't explain that a sugary breakfast like waffles supports none of your nutritional needs, and that your body may suffer with organ system complications like heart disease as a result of frequently heightened blood sugar. They are selling a product to make a profit, so remember that when you select your food.

The placement of every product on a store shelf is part of advertising design. In a commercial, every smiling face serving breakfast food is an actor. Remember that drinking chocolate milk for breakfast will not make you skinny– chocolate milk is a sugary drink that will make you fat. Generally, food that is advertised on TV is likely harmful to your health.[24] I know this to be true. Make your own food or go somewhere where you know who is preparing your meals. Don't ever eat chemicals. Always consider what you need in a day and then give yourself exactly that. Waffles, even 90-calorie waffles, are nothing but cake shaped like a waffle– they are never a breakfast and always a dessert. If I were to own a restaurant, I would place waffles only on the dessert menu and never on the breakfast menu, so everyone would know exactly what they were ordering.

Always be prepared. If you are running from place to place and get hungry, and you have fruit or nuts already in the car, the problem will be solved. Serve yourself with love. Serve your family with love. Love is not found in junk food, love is in real food because real food will set yourself and your family up for the day ahead, armed with nutritional information that will serve their needs.

My love extends from me to you in frank language. I aim to serve you with facts and truths that are meant to educate and inform you. You can take this information anywhere in the world and apply it to any type of person and you will get the same results. If your body only gets junk food, it will respond with illness and fatigue. In contrast, if the body gets mostly nutritious food, it will respond with vitality and vigor.

Become Health Beautiful

Create an environment where healthy food choices can thrive. Going to a health coach to learn about where you are in your life and what keeps you in a place that does not feel good is a terrific step towards gaining control of your health. Seeing another doctor who gives you yet another medication will not serve you at this time.

I used to see a nurse practitioner whose office was always packed because she took over the care of many patients that could not get an appointment with the doctor, and eventually another nurse practitioner had to take over her overflow of clientele. She is lovely and knowledgeable about a lot of things, but nutrition is not one of them. The medical education that most physicians and nurses receive does not typically include a focus on nutrition. This particular NP told me and my husband that there is nothing wrong with eating pizza. As far as I'm concerned and according to my own expertise, yes, there is plenty wrong with pizza. Her advice does one thing for sure– it keeps her office packed and her clients sick.

I like to joke about how her entire office is very liberal with their prescription pad. The doctors and nurses have all asked me what kind of prescription I was there for. I was incredulous when faced with that question. I told her that I am not the doctor, and frankly, I don't want any prescriptions. I want to feel great. Feeling great does not seem like an option for some people. They assume that aging and medication go hand in hand. After taking control of my own life, I can assure you that aging and medication do not need to be inseparable partners. You can feel amazing as you age. You can overcome your tendencies towards sickness and you don't need a doctor's office to make it happen. The first step is clearing your head of all of your thoughts about diet and weight loss. Wipe away your past influences and give yourself a new and powerful goal.

- I will become a Health Beautiful person.
- I will enjoy restful sleep and energetic days.
- I won't feel depressed about my body because I will be physically healthy
- I will enjoy the satisfaction that real food provides to meet my needs.
- I understand that food is fuel and information. My choice of food makes my body beautiful.
- I live pain-free because I am so healthy.
- My family benefits from the balance and stability that good health provides them.
- My kids succeed in school because I have given them every opportunity for good health, which will help them to make their way in a demanding world.
- My partner and I are intimately connected again, now that we are healthy.
- My husband survived potentially tragic dangers because he is so healthy otherwise.
- I think clearly and can enjoy a career that I love with a clear head.
- My hormones are in balance as a result of my clean food choices.
- I use food as a tool to achieve and maintain amazing health.
- I have control over my life because I am not addicted to sugar anymore.
- I have more money because I no longer need to make doctor visits and buy medication for ailments that I can control with my healthy food choices.
- I am in control of my health because I instinctually serve my needs with the highest quality food.
- I crave food that serves my needs.
- I am clear about my needs and how to serve them to keep my dreams alive.

- I look amazing.
- I feel incredible.

Find a few goals that appeal to your true desires. Don't let my voice drown out your voice. What I mean by this is that only you can decide your purpose and the worth of your own future. I am here to offer support and remind you of these goals. I offer the reality of how food affects your body, and I am here to point out when advertisements have clouded your instincts. What I want for you is a feeling of accomplishment, and a feeling of value in your life. I want for you to have a clear connection with your food and your health. I want this for your family as well.

My Wish for Your Health

My goal is to teach the world that understanding food is simple. Food is information, and depending on what kind of food you ingest, your body receives different information. Feed the body cake and the body will read "sugar" and various functions will occur. Feed the body vitamin-rich food and the body will read "vitamins" and respond accordingly. Even when you are in a rush and taxed with many things, your body will still read cake as "sugar" and vitamin-rich food as "information."

Your body works at its best when it is provided with simple real food, and struggles with illness and complications when it is fed processed food. All of the excuses and justifications that you might tell yourself and your family about why convenience is the only option right now do not change how your body will react to poor quality food. You can have convenience and good food at the same time. You just need to open your mind, educate yourself and rethink how you prepare your food.

Selecting healthy food over advertised food will serve your needs. That is why, when you are in a rush and hungry, you need to have a stash of healthy food in the car to hold everyone over until you can all make good choices that serve your nutritional needs, not just impulsive ones. Getting hungry and being unprepared sets you up for failure. Eat before you go anywhere. Never let the kids leave the house hungry. Keeping nuts and fruit in the car allows you to stave off your hunger until you can get to real and beneficial food.

Know your needs and the schedule that your life demands of you. If you work late on Tuesdays, you need to have dinner already prepared for that night on Monday. You can pick up very healthy choices everywhere. Make some rules for your wellbeing and declare that you will never eat fast food. It's as simple as that. Just say, "I will not let that junk pass my lips," and keep that promise to yourself. Give yourself the value that you command and serve yourself only the very best quality food possible. Decide that your family and yourself are worthy of such demands. Refocus on your health rather than your weight and you will automatically raise your quality of living. Your Health Beautiful body is waiting for you to welcome it into your life.

A Sweet Sit-Down

Making an occasional indulgence a regular part of your life can be very beneficial to your overall success. Sugary sweet foods can be very satisfying when respected and indulged in responsibly. Carving out time to make a chocolate treat from scratch or splitting a brownie with a loved one over a cup of tea is a wonderful experience, and I do this with my loved ones all the time. By creating a ceremonial celebration around such indulgences and using only the highest quality food when doing so, you will create a rewarding and fun experience.

In a Health Beautiful life there is room for a perfectly wonderful, special little something every once in a while.

Generations of Healthy Support

Grandparents and other close relatives that spend time with your family need to respect the fact that certain parents don't give their kids lollipops, and likewise, adult children need to listen when their parents say that the food they are giving their grandkids is junk. As your immediate family begins to select healthier food and eat with care, let the people who are in your close circle know what you are doing. Ask for their loving support in your decisions to be healthy. Offer your support for them and their needs as well.

Ask grandparents and other close relatives to leave the lollipops and cookies at home. Insist that they don't stop at fast food places with your kids. In turn, listen to the wisdom they have to offer you about nutrition and their own needs. Don't be defensive or judgmental about their choices, but be firm when it comes to your new nutritional food standards. When your mother-in-law tells you not to bring boxed mac'n'cheese to a family get-together or poses opposition to your fast food runs with your kids, listen. They are in love with your kids and want them to be healthy, too. If they oppose your choice to practice Meatless Monday, explain your reasons and describe the success that you have achieved since you have made these changes. I'd prefer a quick but honest discussion on food with a family member over a lifetime of illness caused by giving in to poor eating habits.

For some reason, adults like to give sweet "treats" to little kids. If you step back and observe this practice, you will see that it looks a lot like someone feeding a biscuit to a dog. The conversation about how your kids react, bouncing off the walls after they have sugary treats, must be held. I know that it may be uncomfortable, but if your child is normal or perhaps particularly sensitive, they will likely react to sugar like a ping pong ball bouncing all over the place. We like to see the kids smile with joy, associating the treat with the person who gave it to them and the sweet taste with the emotion behind a sweet gesture. If this practice is not helping your family on their quest for health, you need to ask for the practice to end. Offer healthier alternatives to the loved one and respectfully ask for your child's needs to be honored.

Be the Voice of Reason in the Family

I love you, so I'm telling you that it's time to take control of your family's health.

A convenient stop for Chinese takeout food or a prepackaged dinner on a busy night does have far-reaching consequences for parents and kids. These breaks in the kitchen routine occur all too often, accumulating over a lifetime of processed food that may lead to a long list of unwanted side effects. Poorly nourished children have been shown to display negative behaviors and illnesses. Please take this seriously– this is not a lecture, it is the truth. Someone has to say it out loud.

Be the parent and give your children real food so this won't happen to them. The ingredients in a fast food meal are not only disgusting, they are absurd. The chemicals that are added to these processed foods are never anything that you would add to your own dishes. They are there to heighten flavor where the natural flavor of real food has been stripped away. The preservatives are added to enhance color and maintain shelf life, because you would never consider eating this food in its actual state.

Because real food is taken apart and chemically changed to save companies money, manufacturers have to figure out how to create a piece of food that resembles something appetizing. This is why certain burger places pour their grill smoke out into the air, so that your senses will be stimulated, creating a desire for their food. Have you ever passed a fast food restaurant and smelled the "grilling" of burgers? This carefully engineered aroma is there to entice you to pull in and buy their product. Even if you weren't hungry, there you are, suddenly wanting a burger. This is an active attempt to persuade you to throw aside your good judgment and eat food that you know is bad for you and your family. I mean look, it is cheap and convenient, and you don't even have to get out of your car. All of these convenient stops that we often make in life add up to a very inconvenient, unhealthy existence.

According to scientists in the field of child nutrition, the following are some side effects displayed in children who eat a poor diet.[25,26]

- Poor concentration
- Obesity
- Victims of bullying
- Hormonal imbalances
- Enlarged breasts in girls and boys
- Depression
- Hyperactivity
- Disciplinary problems
- Anger outbursts
- Type 2 diabetes
- Social difficulties
- Unhealthy drops in blood sugar
- Irritability
- Irregular sleep (too much or too little)
- Endocrine disruption
- Autoimmune disorders

The reset

Create a steady flow of nutrition and sprinkle in convenience by finding supermarkets that offer healthy prepared food. Make selections that are healthy such as whole grains, grilled salmon and sautéed vegetables. You may be too busy to make dinner one night, so plan to pick up dinner from places that only serve healthy food. Plan to bring in food from healthy restaurants one or two times per week rather than five or six times each week. For example, *Meatless Monday* can also mean *veggie sushi lunch day*. Plan to order from a great Japanese restaurant rather than bringing home meatball heroes from the pizza place or a takeout burger from the drive through.

- Know what is going onto the plate and how the body reacts to it
- Cultivate a taste for homemade food

Parenting is challenging on every front, yet we still manage to find joy in the role and do it over and over again. The rewards are worth the struggle. Children are put on a stage daily and judged based on their performance. They are ranked among their peers according to social and academic standards. Their social, academic and athletic achievements are measured and judged. The judges are their peers, teachers, coaches, parents and society as a whole. Their worth is gauged according to how well they meet expectations in school and in society.

I look at my boys who are healthy, inside and out. I see beautiful, strong, capable, intelligent, thin, kind, even tempered, and highly adaptable individuals. Don't get me wrong, they each have their challenges like anyone else. I expect great things from them and put pressure on them to give their very best in everything they do. I also know that we have given them every fighting chance to succeed each day through the healthy food, restful sleep and loving support that my husband and I provide them with. I spend my days thinking about their needs and I am sure to meet them all, starting with food. I'll go through their day ahead of time and check off what they are expected to perform and achieve in their lives.

- Do they have a test? They get eggs and omega-rich smoothies for breakfast.

- Do they play soccer after school? Then they get granola and sunflower seeds for lunch and peanut/seed butter and a banana for a snack.

I know that I am giving my kids everything that they need to face their highly demanding world each day. Like every parent who makes sure that their child has all of their school supplies on the first day of school, I send my kids off with a fresh new set of nutritious meals every day. My job description as their parent and their caregiver states that I am responsible for their wellbeing. That includes nourishment and love. It is hard work, but worthwhile work.

I know it is so much easier to order in at night, to send them with a prepackaged lunch or to have microwaveable snacks in the freezer for after-school hunger pangs. Some parents claim that their kids want snacks with lunch and that is why they send pre-packaged snacks like chips or fruit gummies to school. The problem comes pretty quickly after the snacks are eaten. Kids experience sugar and chemical disruptions that may lead to behavioral issues in class. Unfortunately, the parent is not around all day to see the connection between the snacks and the behavior.

Always set your family out into the world well fed, with proper and usable nutrition. Serve and prepare real food for your family's good health throughout the day. Be conscious of how your family reacts to food. Be observant of their immediate responses and their behavioral responses soon after they eat. Make a note about how long it takes for them to get hungry after a meal. Realize that a hungry kid may be lacking nourishment and a tired kid may not have enough fuel. A disobedient or angry kid may have experienced a severe sugar drop or too many hormonal fluctuations from their food. Kids with acne may have hormonal intestinal disruptions.[27,28]

Look at all of the ingredients in every item found in your child's food for one full day. Make a list and consider whether some of the challenges they experience may stem from what they are eating. If they are eating large amounts of food made with multiple artificial chemicals that act as preservatives, coloring, taste enhancers or stabilizers, then these may be adversely affecting their mental function.

My son told me that many of his friends were eating a popular children's snack bar at school, so I went to check it out at the supermarket. It was advertised as being healthy, so how bad could it be? I quickly discovered that it contains eighty-two ingredients, most of them artificial compounds. (See Appendix B, p. 142.)

When you prepare your own food rather than relying on pre-packaged food, you are able to automatically remove the majority of the chemical ingredients that your family ingests regularly. The simpler your food, the easier it is for your body to use that food for fuel, or to process the vitamins and minerals. If your body does not need to work as hard to access its nourishment, it will work better. It is that simple. The less processed your food is, the fewer demands it will have on the body. The fewer demands put on the body, the more efficiently it works. This is basic biology. To achieve ease in digestion and absorption of good nutrition, one simply needs to consume real, whole, natural food. Food found in the produce section, not the snack and frozen food sections of the supermarket. The items described on the box may be misleading. See Appendix A (p. 140) to discover what is in your own pantry at home.

You are set up for information to come in and energy to go out; any interruption to the process results in stress on the body, and inflammation and illness occur. This is why the body heals so rapidly and this is why we can rely on our heart to beat involuntarily– it is designed to pump our blood continuously, as long as there are no interruptions. Healthy food selection for your family works in a similar way. Your kids will be able to do their jobs as long as they have the proper fuel and there are no interruptions to their metabolic processes.

At times, I find the job of being a parent very demanding. I sometimes think about how much harder and more demanding it would be for my children to have success in their day if I didn't follow through on my end. That is why I do what I do for them, every day.

I do have help. My husband is an important member of our family team. He puts in his share. He will make the food when I have to leave early for work. He will hit the grocery store on his way home or go out late at night to do the shopping, which he prefers since no one is in the supermarket, just fully stocked shelves and him. He sets the table and washes the dishes. He goes to work and still folds laundry. We do it all together because we have a particular mindset about food and nutrition, the same way that some people have a belief in religion.

Someone that I respect highly recently brought up the fact that so many couples have discussions about their core beliefs and marital responsibilities; however, food is rarely a topic of concern. It is odd to me that this could be the case. Many of the problems that my clients deal with have to do with food, kids, and responsibilities at home. The mom wants to make diet changes and the dad continues to bring home bags of chips. Dad is cooking and making healthy meals and Mom is picking up takeout. Having a junk food junkie in the house who does not respect the person who is trying to live a healthy life puts unfair burdens on the family. I often hear from people that they try to eat healthy food but their husband or kids buy or try to make them buy cakes, cookies, pizza, or fast food.

Perhaps you can identify with this scenario. It is a Saturday afternoon. The family is in between two games, one for each child. Everyone needs lunch and there is no time to go home. Someone suggests burgers and everyone says okay, but Mom has been eating like a bird all week, struggling to get rid of her belly fat and fit back into her jeans from last year (she wouldn't dare think about her jeans from two years ago, because that is just way too hard to do).

Here she is, hungry, rushed, and feeling pressured by the family to get unhealthy food. She feels pressure to go along with the family and decides she can just make it up later at the gym. She won't fit into her jeans like she wanted to, and will think that she needs to go to the gym and double her workout, but won't have the time or energy to do it until Monday during work. So, she gives up for the rest of the weekend and indulges in food that does not serve her or her family for the rest of the weekend. Then, Monday comes around and she starts her white-knuckled approach to depriving herself, mixed in with mental struggles to control her calories and burn it off before next Saturday comes around.

Your family wants you to be at your best. They depend on you and don't want to experience your deterioration into illness. They need you to be healthy, happy and well. Many people who are struggling with their family's resistance to change are really struggling with their own resistance to change. It is easy to blame the situation on whiny kids or spouses who don't listen, but if your own heart is not in it, you will never make the changes necessary to experience success. Honesty is the first step in getting your family healthy. This means honesty about how the food that you eat is making you sick, and how it is causing difficulties in your life. Consider all of the reasons why you desire great health. Know each of your family members' reasons for getting healthy. Every person will have different motivations, but every path looks quite similar as it approaches that ultimate healthy state.

As your family gets to understand each other's reasons for wanting to be healthy, you can offer loving support to each member. As one person becomes successful, the others will follow. If one person is looking to improve their work performance, a loving supportive gesture is to offer them an omega-rich smoothie along with their breakfast. If another is having difficulty with giving up added sugar, putting out bowls of berries in the middle of the day is incredibly helpful for distracting them from those cravings. Accountability for your choices without arrogance or judgment is how a family makes lasting changes in their food habits.

In previous chapters, I wrote about paying attention to your family and how they react to food. If your partner suffers from indigestion after a certain kind of meal or you slip into a food coma after another type of meal, it is a good idea to voice how you feel when this happens and what you observe about them. Bringing attention to your observations without judgment is an honest way to create empathy and understanding of each family member's needs.

Lead with Vitality

In my practice, in one of the first sessions I conduct with my clients, we discuss where they plan to get their support. I know that they will be able to reach their goals quickly and stay there when they have support from their families. I love that my clients talk about food and how it serves their nutritional needs with their spouses and children. Understanding your family's needs, even if they don't acknowledge them themselves, is tremendously helpful for your own success. When you set a goal and accomplish that goal, it becomes contagious– the people around you will want to feel and look as good as you.

No one wants to be sick and no one wants to be in pain. We all want our children to feel their best all the time. We want our partners to be the most beautiful that they can be, inside and out. We want our family members to walk with pride and know that your love and support for their success will be there in the most fundamental ways. Nourishing your family and nourishing yourself with love is an expression of

love for all of them. This kind of love makes your family a Health Beautiful family.

Please let me take a moment to emphasize healthy behavior as a model for healthy children. In our current state, we Americans have more obesity among children and adults than ever in time or across most of the world. It is incredibly distressing to imagine that our children are starting their lives in poor health. We struggle to discourage girls from obsessing over retouched models on magazine covers and then feed those same girls hormone- and chemical-laden processed food. The struggles that they may have with weight may indeed come from their own diets, rather than just being a response to the influence of the media. The same holds true for our boys, who attend classes in school discussing alcohol abuse and saying no to drugs and alcohol, just to head home to parents who drink and eat mindlessly in front of the television.

Commercials during sporting events are geared toward male sports fans (and increasingly to a female audience as well), masterfully creating associations between the sport, beer, and eating poor quality food. This association quickly translates to sporting events at school, where parents sit in the stands, rooting on their kids while eating hot dogs and drinking soda. I can't tell you how many times I have been to a game for my kids where parents were speaking loudly and openly about their hangovers and the drinking they had done the previous night. It is a negative message for kids and it needs to be addressed.

When people find out what I do for a living, they often confess that they feel out of control as a result of alcohol use, and some mention their dependence on medications used to relieve depression and stress. While I am not an alcohol or drug counselor, I am mentioning this worrisome aspect of their lives to point out that the struggles in one area of your life may be caused by your choice of stress-reliever. As a parent and a person who wants you to gain some control in your life and the lives of the people around you, I urge you to look at your actions. Take a moment to honestly examine your life. Are you behaving in a way that you are proud to see reflected in your own children? Do you eat the food that you serve to your kids? Do you treat yourself the way that you want your kids to treat themselves? Asking these very difficult questions may be just what you need to do to turn an out-of-control life into a healthy one with grace and ease.

The pride that a parent feels when their child works for something and is awarded proper recognition for that hard work is immense. The joy that is felt when you can proudly say that you were a significant leader in your child's life, and can be proud of their success because of your guidance, will be better than one might imagine. Begin to gain control of your life through leadership. Lead your family to health, and the high achievements to follow, using nutrition. Decide now to treat your own body with the respect that you want your children to be treated with, and together you will soar.

A Helpful List for Reclaiming Your Health

- Feed your body real food
- Eat vegetables all day and include a large variety of them with each meal
- Plan ahead and eat before you get hungry
- Drink more water than you think you need
- Keep a little dirt in your world
- Avoid anything that is processed
- Set aside time each day to indulge in a small amount of good quality chocolate; make sure it is raw, organic and at least 70% cocoa
- Don't get on the scale
- Never buy food that lists the calorie count on the front label
- Know the original source of everything that you eat
- Only eat the very best that you can get your hands on
- Never ever settle for mediocre, fast, processed or second rate meals
- Treat yourself to good quality natural sleep
- Spoil yourself by including fun exercise in a daily routine
- Sweat for a detox
- Make your circle of friends and family the individuals who love and support you
- Remove clutter from your world, especially your kitchen and bedroom

The Journey to Your Beautiful Health

This book is meant to provide a consciousness-raising education, arming you with the knowledge to wisely select real food that supports your body's nutritional demands. I encourage you to read Appendix A (p. 140) and go through the exercise to discover some of the hidden ingredients in your food. Then get started on your journey toward great health.

Start with pure food cookbooks. I loan cookbooks from my personal collection to clients frequently. I encourage my clients to test new recipes that include new and highly nutritious ingredients in dishes that they will enjoy. The first step towards healthy cooking is substituting the stuff that is causing poor health with food that will enhance good health.

Design a plan with a schedule for when and where you intend to buy your food. My clients soon discover new supermarkets and report back to me about how delightful it is to shop in a place that supports their health. They often talk about how exciting it is to try new foods and how nice it is to shop in pleasant markets rather than crowded, overstocked and overwhelming "food" warehouses. Keep an eye out for healthy markets where you can experiment with new foods. By switching to a healthy supermarket you've altered your environment, which will aid you in forming new habits surrounding healthy eating.

If you are seriously pressed for time, I recommend starting in the healthy aisle of your current market. All of the big chains have these kinds of aisles, but be aware that they generally offer a very limited selection. Be sure to uphold the previously mentioned guidelines– no processed food, and select foods that serve your nutritional needs.

A funny thing happened recently to one of my clients. She was looking for whole, organic, plain yogurt with no added sugar. I had warned her that this is not an easy product to find at mainstream supermarkets. She found herself staring at a wall of yogurt selections, none of which satisfied her criteria. I can relate, because I cannot fill a cart at that particular market either, since they offer little that meets my needs. As my client has been changing what she eats, she is also changing where she shops. Her food standards are higher and now she meets those demands by shopping in better quality markets.

Organize your week by designing a meal schedule for several days in advance. Plan to purchase four or five days' worth of vegetables and then clean, cook and store them in separate containers, labeling each. Your planning and preparation will reward you– when you get home after a long day to start dinner, much of the prep is already done and cooking time is minimized.

Eat meals that follow guidelines that help you to meet your health goals, such as Meatless Monday or eating vegan all day until dinner (I often do this and my clients find this easy to achieve). These are just two examples of the types of guidelines that I am suggesting. I also encourage a corn- and corn byproduct-free household. This will eliminate almost all poor quality food from your pantry.

These are the basics for good health that can work for everyone, no matter your ailments or your goals. Every person is very different in what specifically works best for their needs. Leading a vegan lifestyle will not serve the needs of a person who thrives on lean meat. Likewise, giving food based on a paleo diet to a person who is intolerant of red meat is counterproductive to their success.

A nutritional counselor listens to your specific needs. I analyze what you want to achieve and together we decipher how you can meet your goals by satisfying your nutrition. We introduce and incorporate food that is most beneficial to your symptoms of illness and work to change those symptoms into a healthy existence.

For example, one client that I worked with needed to remove red meat from her diet in order to absorb iron more efficiently. Through our conversations and my focused attention on her entire body and all of her symptoms, I was able to guide her naturally and safely towards health. Even though she was anemic, her meat-heavy diet was creating obstructions in her digestive system that did not allow for proper blood flow and proper absorption of minerals. Once we got her onto a healthy vegetarian meal plan, her iron levels quickly normalized. She gained energy and got healthy color back in her skin. Her digestion became regular and she lost weight. Her entire life changed for the better.

People in her life had suggested that she should eat red meat because it contains iron (so do Swiss chard, broccoli, kale, etc.) It took a complete evaluation of all aspects of her lifestyle to identify the cause and correct her illnesses. She was able to create a happier life for herself because of her newly found control over her symptoms.

As her nutritional counselor, I had to get the whole story. She needed to regulate her digestion and then her mineral absorption could resume. That is the sort of life-changing relationship a nutrition coach can have with her clients. The success that a person has in making improvements to their health will develop from listening and applying personalized solutions to their individual needs.

Side Rant: Don't let people who don't know what they are talking about advise you on nutrition. A lot of diet programs and vitamin sales programs are based on hype and profit. Too many people assume that one little tidbit of information applies to every person on the planet. That is how people end up sick and unhealthy. Please, I beg you to leave the nutritional advice to the nutritional experts and let all others carry little weight in your quest for great health.

Taking control of your nutrition, evaluating every aspect of your lifestyle, and striving for balance in places that are not in harmony with the rest of your life will bring you happiness. Feeling calm and educated about how you do the most basic maintenance in your life–providing nourishment–will empower you by creating confidence. You will find confidence in understanding how great food will support your days and how junk and other foods adversely affect your health. Once you can live with a rhythm of health, your whole world opens to rewarding activities that bring you joy. When you no longer have to go to bed exhausted, or you no longer have to take digestive aids just to get through your meals, you are free. With freedom from ailments, a sense of calm and joyfulness takes over.

I encourage you to set your goals in a way that enables you to visualize yourself in a place where your health is perfect. In your vision, you rely on your body to resist disease and recover from illness. You see yourself living the life that you want to live because you have taken control of your health. Controlling your health means giving yourself real food with real results that you can relate to throughout your day. Your new healthy self understands what your body wants and what your body needs. You understand that a 90/10 lifestyle is the way to achieve balance in all aspects of your beautiful life. You understand and know in your head and in your heart that you give yourself and your family love through Health Beautiful living. You are not a slave to the big food industry, you are an educated individual who has confidence in your instincts for what tastes good and what feels good. You have become a person who can honestly say, "I feel great today." You get to say this every day. You are a Health Beautiful person.

You have already begun your Health Beautiful makeover. You consciously made the decision to seek out and read a book on the topic, learning how to nourish your beautiful body. Skipping fast food restaurants and making your own food at home will be the way to ensure that you and your family get the best ingredients possible. Keep your standards elevated when it comes to your food. I encourage you to raise your standards when it comes to all of your basic needs. Your home setting is most comforting when it is free of clutter and when natural light and healthy cooking are priorities. Engaging in a dialogue with your family members about where you stand on food and how your health and their health is your priority creates a fundamental moral ground that you won't falter from.

Resisting the big box stores and choosing your valuable personal time instead has greater significance than saving a few dollars and wasting your time in a warehouse of "food." Take the time to engage in loving support and gentle reminders to your family about how food affects their wellness, and how their needs are more important than the impulses of a crowd or the influences of advertising. Love yourself enough to not judge yourself harshly. Keep a good sense of how your life is enhanced with food and leave the struggles of maintaining a diet in the past. Your appreciation

for real food and delivering it to suit your needs will be a confidence builder.

Forget the diet and welcome the goodness of nutritionally packed food. Pay attention to what you need and how you will meet those needs all week long. Prepare your body with nutrition the way you expect your children to prepare for an exam at school. Gain control of your life through consistent nutritional choices that will allow you to live the life you want to live. Give yourself the boost you deserve to live your life with vibrancy, free from illness. Find motivation that stirs excitement in you for eating well and living well. Include support such as a nutritional counselor who can help to guide you towards your goals. Tap into your family's love to offer and receive support. They love you and want you to be a competent, confident individual.

Congratulations, this is your journey towards living Health Beautifully.

Appendix A

Compare the ingredient lists of what you buy to what you cook at home

This is an exercise to identify what you and your family are eating. There are many chemicals and additives that will startle you when you take a closer look at your food. You will likely discover why you feel so run down or why you cannot lose weight and what keeps your kids from having energy. As you examine these ingredients, ask what they actually are and why they were included. Question if they are necessary. Would you really purchase all of these ingredients and include them in your home-cooked meals? Finally, ask how these ingredients serve you. If they don't serve your nutritional needs, ask who they do serve.

Take the ingredient challenge

Take one day in your life and list all of the ingredients that you consume for the entire day. Do the same for your children and spouse. Knowing exactly what is going into your body is essential to understanding how the food you are eating affects you.

Be honest. As hard as it may be to face the reality of what is in your food, and the more honest that you are being with yourself, the easier it will be to reach your goals of leading a Health Beautiful life. I encounter many people in my practice who will leave certain foods off of their lists because they are ashamed to admit to them. This is not a time for judgment. To make real changes, you need to be honest now.

Be careful not to leave anything off your list, especially if you are a muncher or snacker– there is a chance that you ate something quickly and forgot to add it to your list. Looking around the pantry will cue you in to some foods that you need to add to your list that you may have forgotten.

Don't judge yourself too harshly. You are going through this exercise to bring awareness to what is going into your body and how you are affected by that food. Taking action in this exercise will only make you better at being your best.

Use your phone to snap pictures of the ingredient lists, and then compile them on your computer. Cross-reference the ingredients with what exactly they are and why each item would be added to your food. I find that there are some ingredients that people accept as okay because they see them in everything they eat. Those common ingredients are too often the very additives that may be causing illness.

Don't forget to list spices and sauces, too. Sauce mixes and flavor enhancers like seasoning mix are very important to this list. For example, taco seasoning mix and mayonnaise contain more ingredients than you might think. Take a moment to include these added ingredients on your list.

Try to write the ingredients out in longhand. There are so many additives in so many food products that you may get exhausted and tire quickly of writing them down on paper. This is a good thing. Now consider the effect these additives have on your body. How do several different variations of corn syrup affect your pancreas? How do yellow #2 and blue #7 affect your kids' scholastic abilities? When I do this with children as I am working with families to get their health under control, many are horrified and want to know why a company would add ingredients to their food that are potentially harmful. It can be very emotional for the family to recognize what they have been doing to themselves. Be strong. You have the ability to make changes. Your food does not need to be comprised of these long lists.

Appendix B

Actual ingredient list for a popular breakfast cereal bar, copied exactly as shown on the product:

Cereal (crisp rice [rice flour, sugar, barley malt extract, salt, caramel color], whole grain oats, textured soy flour, sugar, oat bran, corn starch, modified corn starch, honey, brown sugar syrup, salt, calcium carbonate, tripotassium phosphate, canola and/or rice bran oil, zinc and iron [mineral nutrients], vitamin C [sodium ascorbate], a B vitamin [niacinamide], vitamin B6 [pyridoxine hydrochloride], vitamin b2 [riboflavin], natural almond flavor, vitamin B1 [thiamin mononitrate], vitamin A [palmitate], a B vitamin [folic acid], vitamin B12, vitamin D3), Corn Syrup, Milk Filling (sugar, palm kernel oil, lactose, nonfat milk, dried sweetened condensed milk [sugar, milk], partially hydrogenated soybean oil, monoglycerides, soy lecithin, salt, natural and artificial flavor, TBHQ and citric acid added to retain freshness), High Fructose Corn Syrup, Fructose, Maltodextrin, Isolated Soy Protein, Partially Hydrogenated Soybean Oil, Glycerin, Tricalcium Phosphate, Water, Rice Bran and/or Canola Oil, Sorbitol, Soy Lecithin, Caramel and Annatto Extract Color, Sugar, Gelatin, Vitamin C (sodium ascorbate), Natural and Artificial Flavor, Mono and Diglycerides, Iron and Zinc (mineral nutrients), Calcium Carbonate, Salt, Vitamin A (palmitate), a B Vitamin (niacinamide), Vitamin D3, Vitamin B2 (riboflavin), Vitamin B6 (pyridoxine hydrochloride), Vitamin B1 (thiamine mononitrate), a B Vitamin (folic acid), Vitamin B12, BHT and Mixed Tocopherols added to retain freshness.

Would you ever put these ingredients on your shopping list to recreate this popular cereal bar that so many children are eating in your own kitchen?

About the Author

Carissa Kretschmer is a holistic health counselor who helps people to take control of their lives through nutrition. The combination of her extensive science background, certifications in health and nutrition, and continued education at cutting-edge institutions has equipped her with valuable knowledge of how the human body functions in relation to food.

She holds a Bachelor of Science degree from NOVA Southeastern University and a health coaching certificate from the Institute of Integrative Nutrition.

Besides being an involved mother to her two boys, most of Carissa's interests and activities revolve around health and nutrition. She runs a successful counseling practice in Huntington, NY. In her spare time, she cultivates a thriving vegetable garden that provides an endless supply of fresh ingredients for her kitchen and she enjoys cooking fabulous meals, ranging from the simple to the elaborate. Exercise is at the center of Carissa's day, whether she's taking challenging classes at the gym or going on a hike with her loyal Lab.

Contact Carissa via email at

carissa@hbhealthcoaching.com

or visit www.BeHealthBeautiful.com.

Footnotes

---

[1] Hyman, Mark. "5 Clues You Are Addicted to Sugar." Nov. 21, 2014. <http://drhyman.com/blog/2013/06/27/5-clues-you-are-addicted-to-sugar/>.

[2] Vahle-Hinz, T., E. Bamberg, J. Dettmers, N. Friedrich and M. Keller. "Effects of work stress on work-related rumination, restful sleep, and nocturnal heart rate variability experienced on workdays and weekends." *Journal of Occupational Health Psychology.* Apr 19, 2014. Vol. 2, pp. 217-30.

[3] National Institute of Environmental Health Sciences. "Endocrine Disruptors." May 2010. <http://www.niehs.nih.gov/health/materials/ endocrine_disruptors_508.pdf>.

[4] Armstrong, M. J., L. A. Adams, A. Canbay and W. K. Syn. "Extrahepatic complications of nonalcoholic fatty liver disease." *Hepatology.* Mar 2014 Vol. 59, no. 3, pp. 1174-97.

[5] *The Blood Sugar Solution: The UltraHealthy Program for Losing Weight, Preventing Disease, and Feeling Great Now!* Little, Brown and Company. 2012.

[6] Centers for Disease Control and Prevention. "Childhood Obesity Facts." Dec 11, 2014. <http://www.cdc.gov/HealthyYouth/obesity/facts.htm>.

[7] Strawbridge, Holly. "Artificial sweeteners: sugar-free, but at what cost?" *Harvard Health Blog.* July 16, 2012. <http://www.health.harvard.edu/ blog/artificial-sweeteners-sugar-free-but-at-what-cost-201207165030>.

[8] Seinfeld, Jerry. *The Tonight Show.* Dec 23, 2014. <http://videosift. com/video/Jerry-Seinfeld-The-Tonight-Show-12-23-14>.

[9] U.S. Food and Drug Administration. "Guidance for Industry: A Food Labeling Guide." Jan 2013. <http://www.fda.gov/Food/Guidance Regulation/GuidanceDocumentsRegulatoryInformation/LabelingNutrition/ucm0649 28.htm>.

[10] Weil, Andrew. *Spontaneous Healing : How to Discover and Embrace Your Body's Natural Ability to Maintain and Heal Itself.* New York: Random House. 2000.

[11] Mace, T. A., L. Zhong, C. Kilpatrick, E. Zynda, C. T. Lee, M. Capitano, H. Minderman and E. A. Repasky. "Differentiation of CD8+ T cells into effector cells is enhanced by physiological range hyperthermia." *Journal of Leukocyte Biology.* 2011. Vol. 90, no. 5, p. 951.

[12] Perez-Cobas, A. E., M. J. Gosalbes, A. Friedrichs, H. Knecht, A. Artacho, et al. "Gut microbiota disturbance during antibiotic therapy: a multi-omic approach." *Gut.* 2012.

[13] Savage, D.C. "Microbial ecology of the gastrointestinal tract." *Annual Review of Microbiology.* 1977. Vol. 3, p. 107-33.

[14] Blaser, M.J., M. G. Dominguez-Bello, M. Contreras, M. Magris, G. Hidalgo, I. Estrada, Z. Gao, J. C. Clemente, E. K. Costello and R. Knight. "Distinct cutaneous bacterial assemblages in a sampling of South American Amerindians and US residents." Jan 2013. Vol. 7, no. 1, pp. 85-95.

[15] Ravel, J., M. J. Blaser, J. Braun, E. Brown, F. D. Bushman, et al. "Human Microbiome Science: Vision for the Future." From a lecture series held at the Bethesda North Mariott Hotel and Conference Center. Bethesda, MD. July 24-26, 2013. <http://www.microbiomejournal.com/content/2/1/16>.

[16] Savage, D.C. "Microbial ecology of the gastrointestinal tract." *Annual Review of Microbiology.* 1977. Vol. 3, pp. 107-33.

[17] Looft, T. and H. K. Allen. "Collateral effects of antibiotics on mammalian gut microbiomes." *Gut Microbes.* Sep 2012. Vol. 3, no. 5, p. 463.

[18] Sonnenburg, E.D., H. Zheng, P. Joglekar, S. K. Higginbottom, S. J. Firbank, D. N. Bolam, and J. L. Sonnenburg. "Specificity of polysaccharide use in intestinal bacteroides species determines diet-induced microbiota alterations." *Cell.* 2010. Vol. 141, no. 7, pp. 1241-52.

[19] Blaser, M.J., M. G. Dominguez-Bello, M. Contreras, M. Magris, G. Hidalgo, I. Estrada, Z. Gao, J. C. Clemente, E. K. Costello, and R. Knight. "Distinct cutaneous bacterial assemblages in a sampling of South American Amerindians and US residents." Jan 2013. Vol. 7, no. 1, pp. 85-95.

[20] Madara, J. "Building an intestine–architectural contributions of commensal bacteria." *New England Journal of Medicine*. 2004. Vol. 351, no. 16, pp. 1685–1686.

[21] See: The Human Microbiome Project Collection. <http://www.ploscollections.org/article/browseIssue.action?issue=info:doi/10.1371/issue.pcol.v01.i13>

[22] Rippe, James M. and Penny M. Kris Etherton. "Fructose, Sucrose, and High Fructose Corn Syrup: Modern Scientific Findings and Health Implications." *Advanced Nutrition*. September 2012. Vol. 3, pp. 739-740.

[23] Lenoir, M., F. Serre, L. Cantin and S. H. Ahmed. "Intense sweetness surpasses cocaine reward." Aug 2007. Vol. 2, no. 9, p. 698.

[24] Mink, M., A. Evans, C. G. Moore, K. S. Calderon and S. Deger. "Nutritional imbalance endorsed by televised food advertisements." *Journal of the American Dietetic Association*. Jun 2010. Vol. 110, no. 6, pp. 904-10.

[25] Daniels, S. R., D. K. Arnett, R. H. Eckel, S. S. Gidding, L. L. Hayman, et al. "Overweight in children and adolescents: pathophysiology, consequences, prevention, and treatment." *Circulation*. Apr 2005. Vol. 111, no. 15, pp. 1999-2012.

[26] Varela-Moreiras, G. "Controlling obesity: what should be changed?" *International Journal of Vitamin and Nutrition Research*. Jul 2006. Vol. 76, no. 4, pp. 262-8.

[27] Harrist, A. W., L. Hubbs-Tait, G. L. Topham, L. H. Shriver and M. C. Page. "Emotion regulation is related to children's emotional and external eating." *Journal of Developmental and Behavioral Pediatrics*. Oct 2013. Vol. 34, no. 8, pp. 557-65.

[28] Burris, J., W. Rietkerk and K. Woolf. "Relationships of self-reported dietary factors and perceived acne severity in a cohort of New York young adults." *Journal of the Academy of Nutrition and Dietetics*. Mar 2014. Vol. 114, no. 3, pp. 384-92.

9 781508 985532